BOOKS IN A NUTSHELL

TOPIC EDITION

MEDICAL/FOOD/PLANTS

KEY POINTS FROM NON-FICTION BOOKS

31 BOOKS ON MEDICAL

13 BOOKS ON FOOD

7 BOOKS ON PLANTS

STEPHEN S. BATTAGLIA

INTRODUCTION

This is one of five "Books In A NutShell" Topic Edition. Each book includes key points in a number of non-fiction books on a specific topic. As an added help, included prior to each book's facts listing is a synopsis to guide you to the contents of each book. All books are available on Amazon in paperback from, e-book delivered to your kindle, or other sources.

I am sure there are times that you wish you could remember facts about a topic. This book should help you as it includes key and interesting points on various subjects. Each book contains a number of pages of key facts. You will find that it is easier to remember facts when they are grouped together and can be reread quickly to be imprinted on your brain cells. As we age this can be of great help. It is difficult to rummage through a book just to find those facts you knew were there, but it would take too much time to locate them. Now this book makes that much easier. As an example, before going to that financial meeting quickly browse the FINANCE, MONEY and ECONOMIC section in book Volume 2 for some prominent information to be able to show your smarts at that meeting or interview.

Remember the items included are only what I thought were interesting points in the book. They are not all inclusive and it is not a summary of the book. Most of the items were taken directly from the book with little if any changes. Should you desire more in-depth information on any of the books, they can always be purchased. So read on and keep this book handy. Use it like a reference book for easy referral of hard facts on various topics.

MEDICAL SECTION

1. An Introduction to Human Evolutionary Anatomy
by Chris Dean

Synopsis: Information and review of elements of the human body.

1. Taxon- a group of organisms at any level of hierarchy.
2. Trabeculae or a spongy region of a bone is 25% renewed every year.
3. The mandible and the cranium together are known as the skull.
4. The temporal bones called because graying hair at the temples was the first signs of ageing.
5. Teeth- 32 in total and four muscles for moving the mouth. Most can open our mouths to about three-fingers between upper and lower teeth.
6. Bulk of all tooth tissue is formed of dentine and the crowns of teeth are covered with a layer of enamel, which is the hardest biologically formed substances known.
7. All teeth pass through three phases: calcification, enamel formation and closure of the apical canal of the root
8. Four types of teeth- incisors, canines, premolars, and molars.
9. Interior of the cranial cavity is divided into three cranial fossae. The intracranial cavity is divided into compartments by tracts of fibrous dura mater and protect the brain.
10. Beneath and surrounded by the dura mater are the arachnoid and the pia mater all three known as the meninges of the brain.
11. The brain is regulated to about 37deg. C. or 98.6 F.
12. A neuron consists of a cell body and processes known as dendrites and conveys information to the cell body.
13. Tissues of the central nervous system are composed of either grey matter or white matter. Gray matter contains cell bodies and white matter contains axons, which appear white to the naked eye.
14. Motor nerve fibers are nerves that leave the brain via the spinal cord which bring about movements. Sensory nerves refer to taste, vision, hearing or smell and enter the brain as cranial nerves.
15. Cerebral cortex is divided into – frontal, parietal, temporal and occipital lobes.
16. Temporal lobes are concerned with watching and hearing as music.

17. Hippocampus part of the limbic system and is associated with memory

18. Patients with lesions of the cerebellum commonly experience slurring of their speech, and tremors.

19. Net weight of the human head is normally 5.4% of the body weight and is less in animals.

20. Larynx, a series of cartilages, is a valve like structure that guards the opening into the trachea or windpipe.

21. In humans there are 33 vertebras

22. Sternum, meaning solid or hard, are bones of the upper chest and divided into three sections.

23. In the hand there are 27 bones which 14 are bones of the fingers

24. Patella is the large bone of the knee in front of the femur muscle.

25. The foot is made up of 26 small bones including 7 ankle or tarsal bones.

26. Leg bones- femur (the largest), tibia, and the fibula.

27. The gluteus maximus is the extensor of the hip and the largest muscle of the rump or buttock.

2. Another Day in the Frontal Lobe by Katrina Firlik

Synopsis: A review of the brain and its functions.

1. The brain makes up about 80% of the intracranial contents. The other 20% is split between blood and cerebrospinal fluid.

2. Neurological organizations – AANS (American Assoc. of Neurological Surgeons) and CNS (Congress of Neurological Surgeons).

3. Dr.'s Watson and Crick discovered DNA in early 1950's.

4. Total human blood volume is about 5 liters (5.3 quarts- or 2.6 gallons or about 21.6# at 8.33 #/gal.

5. To work in the brain a hole the size of a nickel is drilled with a special tool, a perforator, that drills and stops when you are through the bone.

6. Benign tumors-meningioma's- arise from the outer covering of the brain and cause problems by indenting into the brain or pushing it aside. True tumors of the brain tissue, known as gliomas, are the most feared and known as primary brain tumors- metastases that originate from cancer outside the brain.

7. Cell death is called necrosis. Water on the brain is called hydrocephalus.

8. The cerebrospinal fluid surrounds the brain and fills four ventricles in the brain. It is produced and absorbed at the rate of about 450cc per day about ½ liter.

3. Brandwashed by Martin Lindstrom

Synopsis: How items we eat and drugs we take effect our body.

1. By the age of 7 brand and product preferences are embedded in their minds.

2. Foods are primed in our minds by about 4 years old.

3. 53% of adults and 56% of teens used brands from their childhood.

4. Viruses are spread via tiny droplets in the air via sneezed or coughed by infected people.

5. Fear of failure rather than promise of success drives consumers. Promise of success tends to paralyze us.

6. Ads work because they induce fear and guilt

7. Averting gazes are associated with shame and social isolation while straight ahead gaze is a sign of confidence and connectedness.

8. Domestic sales of prescription drugs are about $236 billion.

9. How we get hooked on a brand: routine stage of daily use and emotional need.

10. Caffeine restricts the blood vessels in our brains.

11. Lip balms especially Carmex use phenol and salicylic acid that tears away at tissue like corns and calluses. Actually, ends up drying the lips and require more use and stops the lips from excreting necessary oils.

12. In Europe more men wear fragrance than American females. When women choose a product 80% is emotional and 20% is rational.

13. A study showed that our brains are not fully matured until age of 24.

14. Less confidence or self-esteem one has the more they are dependent on brands.

15. Mentioning time in an ad is more likely to be successful.

16. Average person carries around 15 loyalty cards.

17. By the age of 2, 92% of American children have a digital footprint.

4. Doctors- Info from a DVD by DR. NULAND

Synopsis: The history of doctors, what they discovered, and some commonly used medical terms.

1. Hippocrates 460 BC- father of medicine. Apollo was the father of healing. In this period doctors believed in the power of the snake. That is why there is a snake on a medical stick.

2. Golden age of Greece was the 3rd century BC. Observed if the individual was sick by viewing- blood, or phlegm- yellow or black. If the Individual had a fever they removed blood. Start of the ethical code in medicine.

3. Galen- 131AD-basic research and determined that acid dissolved food in the stomach, started dissecting parts of the body and determined urine was made in the kidneys.

4. Versalius-1543- first book on anatomy. First school of medicine was in Selorno, Italy in the 6th century. In 1087 the University of Padua, Italy opened for the study of law, medicine and theology. Pope Sixtus IV's 1450 edict was that cadavers could be given to doctors and artists for study. Nothing is to be believed until verified.

5. Harvey 1578- Circulation of the blood, heart bests @ 72x per minute. Start of inductive reasoning. Systole is heart contracting. Diastole is heart at rest. Heart will hold 2 oz. of water. Determined that the heart pumps blood to the body. Malpighi 1621- heart pumps blood to body and capillaries return the blood to the heart.

6. Morgagni 1705- father of physical examination. – Age of enlightenment. He wrote a book on appendix.

7. Hunter 1750- First artificial insemination. The seven-year French & Indian war.

8. Laennec- discovered the stethoscope, (a Greek word- stetho- chest and scope- to observe). In 1816 he first used a rolled-up paper. Cirrhosis of the liver was studied and partially determined its cause.

9. Morton- 1846 anesthesia. Used euphoric ether. Priestly used nitrous oxide in 1772.

10. Virchow1845- start of cell investigation to determine disease. Leukemia is the excess of white cells. Blood clot- thrombus, blood clot that kills is called embolis. There are 200 types of cells and 75 trillion cells.

11. Leister- germ theory -41% of amputees died of infection before antiseptic was discovered.

12. Halstead-1874- John Hopkins Hospital was started with the help of four woman who helped raise $1 million on condition that woman would be admitted and a college degree was required. This led to the admission standards.

13. Hernia is a hole in the abdominal wall. Development of rubber gloves in operating rooms was in the late 1800's.

14. Taussug 1923 development of cardiac transplantation.

15, Blue babies occur when a hole in right ventricle sends unoxygenated blood to the left ventricle. 1950 first heart machine.

16. Discovery of a fungus, cyclosporine, helped to assist a heart transplant to accept a new heart.

5. Herbal Antibiotics by Stephen Buhner

Synopsis: The review of herbs their purpose and their effect on our body both good and bad.

1. Adverse drug reactions are the 4th leading cause of death in the U.S.

2. Per year over 60 million antibiotics are used in the U.S. in 2009 with nearly ½ used on animals.

3. Antibiotics promote exchange of plasmids, which may contain resistances genes. Most water supplies in industrialized countries are contaminated with antibiotics.

4. Triclosan in toothpastes causes bacterial resistance.

5. Testing in 2011 found that 50% of store-bought meat and poultry were contaminated with staph. To kill salmonella bacteria in eggs fry or boil for at least 9 minutes.

6. Flies found to be the main spread of resistant organisms in the general community.

7. The money's not in the cure it is in the medicine. Between 1983 and 2008 investment in antibiotic research development in the US fell by 75%.

8. Within 5 years MRSA will be completely untreatable by antibiotics and its over use. Green tea as well as pomegranate has properties that helps inhibit MRSA.

9. Over 70% of all pathogenic bacteria in hospitals are at least minimally resistant.

10. Herbs that can help infections- ginger, echinacea, juniper berry, licorice, and oregano oil.

11. Some of the main herbs to treat MRSA are: sida, black pepper, usnea, juniper berry, licorice, ginger, honey.

12. Prior to 1977 no reports of resistance in cholera organisms but now common.

13. Top systemic herbal antibiotics: cryptolepis, sida, alchornea, bidens and Artemisia.

14. The herb cryptolepine is cytotoxic and kills cancer cells because it intercalates the DNA by inserting itself between the two DNA ladders.

15. Artemisinin is an antitumor and anti-cancer compound.

16. Top 4 non systemic herbal antibiotics: bebeerines, juniper, honey & usnea

17. Honey- known to resist bacteria on infected skin and wounds. Good for treatment of colds and respiratory infections. Get organic and wildflower if available. Read labels as some include things other than honey as sugar. Good to be cloudy with pollen.

18. Licorice-moderately antibacterial and potently antiviral. The root and leaves are acceptable.

19. Ginger is a synergist, which increases the actions of other herbs and boosting their effectiveness and increases circulation.

20. Reishi is a fairly potent anticancer acting herb. It helps reduces cancer cells.

21. Cold and flu drink: sage, cayenne, wildflower honey, lemon juice,

22. Nasal spray for sinus infections: five drops of each, cryptolipis, bidens, juniper berry and usnea

6. Incognito- "The Secret life of the Brain"
        by David Engieman

Synopsis: Some interesting facts on the brain and how it affected some people.

1. The brain is built of cells- neurons and glia.
2. A neuron has about 10 thousand connections.
3. A brain weighs about 3 pounds.
4. Pitcher Nolan Ryan's fast ball at 100 mph reaches the plate in about 4 tenths of a second.
5. Galileo Galilei on January 10, 1610 observed Jupiter and its moon and thought at first, they were stars.
6. Ptolemy said the center of the universe is the earth. Copernicus said the sun was the center.
7. One third of the brain is devoted to vision.
8. Testosterone in boys produce prominent chin, a larger nose, fuller jaw, growth of muscles and broad shoulders. For females' estrogen produces full lips, full buttocks and growth of breasts.
9. Front brain hemisphere is connected by fibers called corpus callosum. The left hemisphere of the brain is for language.
10. Parkinson's patients when given the drug pramilpexole turned them into gamblers. Parkinson is due to the loss of brain cells dopamine.
11. Roper v. Simmons stated that there was no death penalty for those under 18.
12. Ugly people receive longer sentences than attractive people.
13. Drug use as a teenager increases the development of psychosis as an adult.

7. Musicophilia   by Oliver Sacks

Synopsis: Technical data of music and its effect on individuals.

1. Imagining music stimulates the motor cortex and imagining the action of playing music stimulates the auditory cortex. Musical imagery is even intensified by deafness.
2. Musicians increase the prevalence of hearing loss with music overload in high pitch.

3. The corpus callosum in the brain of professional musicians is inherited and the plenum temporal enlargement indicates absolute pitch.

4. Young children respond to training by ear and imitation of the violin. Brief exposure to classical music can stimulate or enhance mathematical, verbal and visual abilities in children- so called the "Mozart Effect".

5. There are records of striking changes in the left hemisphere of children who have had only a single year of violin training.

6. Absolute pitch is highly dependent on early musical training.

7. Hindu music has 22 note scales.

8. Your inner ear, the cochlea, has 3,500 sterocilia or inner ear hair cells.

9. Impairments of melody usually go with right hemisphere lesions while rhythm involves the left hemisphere and other sub cortical systems including the cerebellum.

10. Amelodia means tune deafness.

11. The path of sound in the ear passes through the eardrum to the tiny bones, ossicles, on either side and on to the snail shaped cochlea with its 3,500 hair cells.

12. Inner ear hair cells although protected by the organ corti can be destroyed by very loud sound.

13. Cerebral right hemisphere is for perceptual skills and the left lobe the development of abstract and verbal powers. The cerebral left hemisphere takes longer to develop.

14. Early musical training, before 6 or 8, is crucial in the development of maintenance of absolute pitch.

15. Speech of words has inflections, intonations tempo, rhythm, and melody.

16. Loss of musical emotion is more common with damage to the right hemisphere of the brain.

8. Tale of the Dueling Neurosurgeons by Sam Kean

Synopsis: A review of the brain and the doctors who originally studied it.

1. Frontal lobes of the brain help us plan, make decisions and set goals. Back or occipital lobes process vision; top of parietal lobes combine vision, hearing, touch and other sensations; side or temporal lobes help produce language.

2. Galen served as a doctor for Roman gladiators and was born in AD 129.

3. Nervous system contains two main types of cells- neurons and glia. Neurons process thoughts while gli, meaning glue, hold neurons in place and provide nutrients to the system.

4. Neurons have branches of dendrites and axons. The axon cables zip information from one gray matter node to another at speeds up to 250 miles per hour.

5. Brain's contains two distinct substances- gray and white matter. Gray matter has a high percentage of neurons and most reside on the brain's surface called the cortex.

6. In July 1900, Gaetano Bresci assassinated King Umberto I of Italy.

7. Nations first execution by electricity occurred in 1890 in Auburn, New York.

8. In 1938, Albert Hofmann in searching for a new drug developed LSD through fungi and tried it in April 1943.

9. Chinese surgeons performed the second face transplant in April 2006 with remarkable results. The first was performed in 2005 to unknown long-term results.

10. Modern nursing began with Florence Nightingale in Crimea during the Franco-Prussian War.

11. Amino Acids are the building blocks of proteins.

12. Anosognosia- inability to recognize illness.

13. Right lobe of the brain controls the left side of the body and the left lobe controls the right side.

14. The brain needs thiamine to make myelin sheaths to build neurotransmitters. Our body needs B1 (thiamine via vegetables, beans or meat) to harvest energy for glucose the end result of digesting carbohydrates.

15. Alcohol prevents the intestines from absorbing thiamine and causes changes inside the brain especially to the glia cells. Without thiamine the glia cannot sop up glutamate and causes neurons to die or excitotoxicity.

16. Lying or continuously fibbing for no obvious reason is known as confabulation.

17. Hippocampus records and stores memories.

18. Largest structures in the brain are the left and right hemisphere lobes.

19. Back of the left hemisphere frontal lobe is known as Broca's area and controls speech production.

20. Parietal lobe handles basic arithmetic.

21. Reading disorder is known as alexia sine agraphia.

22. Darwin studied natural selection.

23. Corpus callosum is where seizures occur.

24, Right brain is for music.

25. Thalamus at the core of the brain receives information and relays it around the body.

9. The Cancer Chronicles; Unblocking Medicine's Deepest Mystery   by George Johnson

Synopsis: A review of cancer its causes and some controllable hints.

1. All mammals have precisely seven vertebrae in their necks. However, birds and amphibians are not bound by this rule as a swan can have 22 to 25.

2. Cancers are combated by antifolates. One helpful dish is sautéed spinach with garlic.

3. Supplements sometimes increase the risk of a disease. As too much of something is a bad thing.

4. Little reason to believe that multi vitamins are helpful unless a person is severely malnourished.

5. Controlled trials have shown that a diet low in fat and high in fiber with fruits and vegetables had much effect or reduced colorectal polyps a precursor to colon cancer.

6. It matters mostly on how much you eat and not what you eat. Actually, excess body fat reduces the chances of premenopausal women getting breast cancer.

7. A study has shown that for women every 4 inches over 5 feet increases the cancer risk by 16%.

8. Vitamin D lowers the odds for colorectal cancer but raises the risk for pancreas cancer.

9. PET stands for Positron Emission Tomography- recondite world of particle physics.

10. For tumors to expand it must find a way to reach into the circulatory system for blood.

11. In the 1920's Hermann Muller got the first hint that cancer is a disease and that X-rays and long exposure to the sun might be responsible for its ability to cause cancer.

12. X-rays by W. Rontgen in 1895 when used on mutated flies either killed them or sterilized them.

13. Paradox: why the cancer-killing rays could also produce cancers, transforming normal cells into malignant ones.

14. Ancient Rome mined uranium from a rock called pitch-blend for its yellow pigment for glass and ceramics. Not until 1896 was their exotic qualities known.

15. Coal tar applied to animals in lab experiments gave them tumors. When people smoke that was the same thing and shown to cause cancer.

16. Mitosis is the process of healthy cells dividing.

17. Scientists began in 1980's discovering anti-oncogenes.

18. P53 slows down the clock so that DNA repair can take place.

19. Hayflick- a normal cell can divide only 50-60 times.

20. Amphibians and planaria regenerate amputated body parts.

21. Human hedgehog gene involved in sprouting of hair from follicles- treatment for baldness.

22. Companies that produced the carcinogenic chemicals also make drugs used for the chemotherapeutic cures.

23. Cancer causes: tobacco 30%, obesity and inactivity 20%, diet about 20%, alcohol 4%, viruses 3%

24. In 1973 Ames showed that carcinogens caused cancer by inducing genetic mutations.

25. Black pepper contains safrole; mushrooms contain hydrazines that have caused cancer in mice. But depend on the quantity taken.

26. Japan leads the world in stomach cancer due to salty fish eaten.

27. Cisplatin known as the penicillin of cancer has the effect of rapidly dividing cells but also a sickening side effect.

28. Doxorubicin operated by interfering with the replication of DNA.

29. Cancer drug adriamycine pushes down your white blood cell count increasing vulnerability to infections. The name comes from the Adriatic Sea.

30. Paclitaxel or Taxol was originally isolated from the bark of the Pacific yew tree.

31. Striking a cancer with combination of different drugs increases the odds of killing it.

32. Mesothelioma is the cancer associated with exposure to asbestos.

33. There are approximately 25,000 genes in a human genome and at least 350 identified as possible cancer genes.

34. In 1928 in St. Mary's Hospital in London, Alexander Fleming discovered penicillin.

35. As much as 50-60% of cancers we didn't have the slightest idea of where it comes from.

36. Sources of cancer: salt- stomach, red and processed meat-colon cancer, but smoking is the strongest for lung cancer.

37. Foods rich in cancer protective chemicals- onion family, cabbage family, vegetables as broccoli, cauliflower, kale, brussel sprouts, peas, tomatoes and deep yellow vegetables and fruits-raisins, prunes, blueberries.

38. Cortisol a stress hormone and melatonin regulate sleep.

39. The cerebellum is the center of muscular control and balance.

40. It is not clear whether screening via annual mammograms does any good and probably does more harm than good.

10. The Folly of Fools: the Logic of Deceit and Self Deception in Human Life by Robert Trivers

Synopsis: Information on the brain and a review of group's control of foreign lands.

1. The more ignorant the individual the more confident he or she maybe.

2. Bias begins early in life. By age three they prefer to play within group members.

3. Power tends to corrupt and absolute power corrupts absolutely.

4. About 1% of bird species is entirely dependent on other species to raise their young as cuckoos.

5. Hippocampus part of the brain is where memories are stored.

6. The mind resists suppression and does the opposite.

7. White matter in the brain nourishes the neurons via the glial cells. Liars have more white matter in the area of the brain involved in deception.

8. Right and left brains are connected by a corpus callosum. Left-brain is the linguistic side.

9. Antidepressants accounts for about 25% of improvement and placebo effect accounts for the remaining 75%. Just believing you are getting something to help is over 1/2 the battle. Across the population- 1/3 very strong, 1/3 somewhat, and 1/3 none on placebo effect.

10. Hypothalamus of the brain is involved in hunger and growth.

11. Every two weeks, roughly the max. life span of white blood cells, the body produces a set of cells greater in volume than 2 grapefruits.

12. For every 1 Degree C increase in body temp we lose about 20% in total body protein or energy loss in sick humans.

13. The more sleep the higher the white blood cell count. Red cells are no part of the immune system.

14. The brain represents about 3% of the body weight but 20% of the energy consumption.

15. Light music mode helps the immune system and health of the body.

16. 100% of stocks change hands every Month and 5 billion are traded per day.

17. With spam 9 out of 10 e-mail messages are junk.

18. Lie detector tests- measures three variables- heart rate, breathing amplitude and galvanic skin response.

19. 45% of airplane accidents occur when a pilot or copilot is flying for the first time.

20. By law an elevator must be built 11 times stronger than required with full load and travel.

21. Harry Truman said "the only thing new under the sun is the history you do not know".

22. Due to the Spanish holocaust of the 1500's the population was reduced to 5% due also to diseases and genocide.

23. The U.S. invaded Nicaragua 13 times in the 20th century turning the contras loose on them in the 1980's.

24. Turkish Government committed genocide against the Armenians, Zionist conquerors ethnic cleansing of 700,000 of Palestinians, the early Americans of the U.S. did the same to the Indians of North America.

25 .In 1920 there were about 80,000 Jews and 700,000 Arabs in Palestine. Israel occupied southern Lebanon from 1982 to 2000 until Hezbollah drove them out.

26. Jewish state in 1947 via the UN mandate the size of Israel was 56% of Palestine and through a war expanded to 78%. 1994 Oslo accord was broken through increase Jewish settlements.

27. Paul Wolfowitz of the Pentagon assured Congress that the war in Iraq would cost about a few billion, and would be paid for with their oil.

28. According to cognitive dissonance theory the greater the cost the greater self-deception.

29. The Black Plague wiped out 1/3 of Europe in the Middle Ages.

30. Religious behavior has a positive correlation with health formulating rules to avoid tobacco, alcohol, and gambling.

11. The Mind's Own Physician by Dalai Lama- Dialogue

Synopsis: Some interesting facts on the brain.

1. Three fundamental elements: responsible behavior, mental collectedness, and development of insightful understanding.

2. There is strong evidence to show musical training can influence the brain. Learning new motor skills helps.

3. Our brain oscillates at the rate of about forty hertz.

4. Stress makes it difficult for the stomach to repair the beginnings of an ulcer.

5. Brain has two systems yin and yang responsible for positive and negative emotions.

6. Buddhist practice consists of three parts: ethics, mind training, and wisdom.
7. Destructive emotions such as anger and fear cause changes in the mind, body, and brain.
8. Three dimension pixels are known as voxels

12. "UNDERSTANDING THE BRAIN"
from Great Courses- DVD #29

Synopsis: A study of music and its effect on individuals.

1. Music is a sequence of tones and its relationships, and is the same for language.
2. Both language and music have rhythm, tempo, and anticipation.
3.   A. Musicians- powered by the left hemisphere
     B. Non-musicians –the right hemisphere is for rhythm and tempo, and left hemisphere is for anticipation.
4. Auditory is processed in the temporal lobe in the mid brain.
5, Amusia- music agnosia is the loss of the ability to appreciate music.
6, Music is a limbic system experience that increases dopamine and endorphins in the brain and all processed in the hippocampus. Some musicians can remember long sequences of music.
7. Music development- early childhood is important and the brain can develop this if exposed in early adulthood.
8. "Music communicates emotional feelings that words cannot."

13. White Bread by Arron Strain

Synopsis: A historical review of bread from early Egypt to current times.

1. Companion- from Latin roots: com- work, and pan – bread.
2. Pharaonic Egypt workers received wages in bread and bread grains.
3. 13th century Britain workers on feudal manors ate 70 to 80% of daily calories in form of bread and cheese. Beer made up most of the rest.

4. By 1950 calories from bread went to 40-60 % of daily calories.

5. Cheap U.S. corn exported by multinational grain traders, subsidized by the U.S. government, displaced a million or more small farmers in Mexico.

6. In 1830 Sylvester Graham named the graham cracker.

7. By 1890, 90% of bread was made at home by woman. By 1930 90% was made by factories.

8. In July 1920 sliced bread was invented.

9. All wheat flour whitens naturally through oxidation as it ages for one to two months. Chemical bleaching is used to whiten the flour with chlorine or nitrogen peroxide gas; some bakers used chalk, boras and alum to whiten dark flour.

10. Court case to charge Lexington Mill and Elevator with selling poisonous ingredients in bread with their bleaching process. Supreme Court ruled that use of the word "may" in the 1906 Pure Food and Drug Act was enough for the Gov. to win the case. Flour then sold as unbleached flour. Previously all commercial flour was treated with chlorine gas or nitrogen.

11. Pro racers ate anti-inflammatory foods as raspberries, ginger and salmon to speed the recovery from injuries. Also ate gluten free foods and were mentally fresh, slept better and performed at a higher level.

12. Grains containing gluten as rye, barley, and sometimes oats. Gluten is added to some foods as ketchup and spices. With increased breeding in wheat, it contains increased gluten levels.

13. Global cholera pandemic reached the U.S. via Canada in 1832. Doctors recommended no meat or white bread and lots of pure water.

14. In 1915 a German battleship on a 255-day voyage with sailors on a diet of white flour, white potatoes, white sugar and red meat died of this diet.

15. Fasting was a weapon for the body to manage microbes from eating.

16. Due to lack of vitamins, the draft board doctors rejected 500,000 out of the 1 million for military service.

17. One half of the TV shows in the 1950's featured cowboys.

18. Pres. Truman mobilized the largest movement of wheat and flour for the war cause in 1946/7. In 1958, 96% of the staple in Greece was U.S. flour or wheat and Turkey followed.

19. 1943 under the Rockefeller Foundation established the Office of Special Studies called Mexican Agriculture Program or MAP. Corn covered 65% of Mexican agriculture land and the main ingredient in their diet. They started using U.S. pesticides, mechanized harvesting and synthetic fertilizer. By 1957 90% of their wheat seeds planted in Mexico were of the industrial varieties.

20. By 2009 whole wheat bread sales topped white.

21. In 1951 Congressional testimony of 17,000 pages on the question of bread "are we eating poisoned bread".

14. Wicked bugs by Amy Stewart

Synopsis: A review of some bugs and other related items.

1. An aphid is a type of insect that we call a bug, an ant is not. Spiders, worms, centipedes, slugs and scorpions are not insects but are arachnids.

2. Columbus's second voyage to the New World was to the island of Hispaniola now Haiti and Dominican Republic.

3. Treatment for malaria is quinine extracted from the bark of the
   S. African cinchona tree.

4. Malaria is from the Italian word for "bad air".

15. The Alzheimer's Prevention Program
by Gary Small, MD and Gigi Vorgan
Keep your brain healthy for the rest of your life

Synopsis: A review of Alzheimer's disease and dementia. Included are helpful suggestions to maintain and improve your brain function.

1. Age is the single greatest risk factor for developing memory loss.

2. To protect the body and mind it is helpful to have: Physical exercise, a nutritious diet, mental stimulation and stress reduction.

3. Science has shown that genetics accounts for only part of our risk for Alzheimer's disease.

4. In 1906 Alois Alzheimer presented the first report on the disease that was later named after him.

5. Alzheimer's disease is a disease attacking the brain cells- a buildup of sticky proteins that caused neurons to misfire, mucking up their signals.

6. Plaques and tangles begin to build up in the brain decades before any symptoms of Alzheimer's emerge.

7. One out of five people carry a common genetic variant known as APOE-4 that has some risk for individuals getting Alzheimer's disease after the age of 65.

8. Eating antioxidant fruits and vegetables to combat Oxidation is a critical component of a diet that protects us from Alzheimer's disease.

9. Drugs such as Motrin a new Alzheimer's preventive or cure have potentially dangerous side effects as elevated blood pressure and possible internal bleeding.

10. People who spend time doing complex mental tasks during midlife decreased their dementia risk by as much as 48 percent.

11. Two tasks that can determine how your brain is functioning:
 Is a baseline assessment of subjective memory (how one perceives one's memory) and objective memory (how one actually performed on a memory test).

12. There are three levels of physical conditioning: aerobic conditioning, strength training, and balance and stability.

13. An Alzheimer's prevention diet involves not only settling on a correct weight but also eating the right kinds of fats, proteins, and carbohydrates.

14. Memory consists of getting information into the brain and retrieving that information later. This involves a complex array of biochemical events, electrical transmissions, and neuronal connections that occur throughout the brain.

15. Scientific evidence shows that practicing basic memory methods sharpens memory capacity, slows related decline and helps maintain peak memory performance.

16. A helpful memory strategy is: LOOK-focus on what you want to recall later, SNAP-form a visual image or sharpshot of the information, CONNECT-create visual associations.

17. Daily brisk walks led to a 40% lower risk of developing Alzheimer's disease or any kind of dementia. Exercise releases endorphins, the body's own natural antidepressant, and serotonin in the brain.

18. Depression can distract us and impair our memory ability. It can also be one of the first symptoms of the onset of Alzheimer's disease in older adults.

19. The smooth, circular movement of cycling not only provides an aerobic challenge, but it can even strengthen knee joints. Swimming offers a great cardiovascular workout and engages almost every major muscle group in the body.

20. Resistance and strength training helps make bones denser and lowers our risk for osteoporosis.

21. Balance and stability training can include: dancing, tai chi or pilates.

22. People who have a lower risk for Alzheimer's disease in a study were those who ate a greater amount of nuts, fish, tomatoes, poultry, vegetables, and fruits. They ate lesser amounts of high-fat dairy products, red meat, and butter.

23. Omega-3 fatty acids from foods like fish (salmon, trout and tuna but not farmed fish) will stabilize mood and diminish depression.

24. Low levels of antioxidants in the blood are associated with memory impairment. Foods high in antioxidants are prunes, blueberries, apples, strawberries, grapes, sweet potatoes, beets, broccoli, cabbage, celery, and raw garlic. This includes fruit or vegetable juices. Antioxidant spices include: oregano, cinnamon, turmeric and parsley.

25. To protect our brains, we need to minimize our intake of omega-67 fats as bacon, lamb chops, butter, most fried foods, as well as corn and vegetable oils. Instead eat wild salmon and eat walnuts as a snack.

26. Our body needs amino acids as building blocks for all proteins to maintain normal body cellular function. You can get these from such items as fish, poultry, eggs, yogurt, cheese and soybeans. They all contain 9 of the 20 amino acids that our body needs.

27. A study showed that light drinkers had a 30% lower risk for dementia when compared to people whom either abstained completely or who overindulged.

28. Moderate drinking of caffeinated coffee was shown to protect the brain and associated with a 65% lower rate of developing Alzheimer's disease.

29. Socially engaged individuals may reduce their risk for dementia by as much as 60%.

30. As we age the right and left-brain hemispheres work together more effectively. The left hemisphere is more analytical and verbal while the right hemisphere is more visual and emotional.

31. Our brains pass information through billions of dendrites. When we don't use our dendrites, they can shrink or atrophy. Brain games aim to stimulate our minds and work out our dendrites to extend their branches.

32. The University College in London suggests that people who delay retirement by several years have better cognitive abilities than those who retire earlier.

33. In a Stanford University study, chronic stress seems to shrink the hippocampus, a brain area that controls memory processing.

34. Cortisol is one of the hormones the body secretes while under stress. Cortisol injections have shown to impair verbal memory ability. However, these impairments were temporary.

35. Getting good night's sleep is important to brain function, as our brain is extremely active during sleep.

36. About 30% of people suffer from insomnia. A few strategies to assist are: stay up during the day, avoid evening liquids, keep a low profile in the evening, avoid caffeine at night, and maintain a regular sleep routine.

37. Drugs have been developed to help brain function and include donepezil, rivastigmine and galantamine.

38. Alzheimer's disease is not just an abnormality of amyloid deposits; many other normal structures and functions are breaking down in an Alzheimer's brain.

39. Symptoms of cognitive loss and depression often become intertwined.

40. Physical conditioning, healthy diet, mental exercise, and stress management can make a difference in how we feel and function now and in the future.

16. THE SLEEP REVOLUTION by Arianna Huffington
   Transforming your life, one night at a time

Synopsis: Some history of sleeping studies, and helpful methods of sleeping, and foods that help or hinder sleep.

1.   In the 1970's, there were only 3 centers in the United States devoted to studying sleep disorders. By 1990, that number had swelled to more than 300 and now it's more than 2,500.

2. Sleep is a time of intense neurological activity- a rich time of memory consolidation brain and neurochemical, cleansing, and cognitive maintenance.

3. Getting by on less than six hours of sleep is one of the biggest factors in job burnout.

4. A lack of melatonin, the hormone that controls our sleep and wake cycles, is linked to higher rates of breast, ovarian, and prostate cancers.

5. While we sleep, the brain is able to get rid of toxins, including proteins that are associated with Alzheimer's disease.

6. Sleep problems are the number-one military disorder when people come back from deployments.

7. Women are the biggest users of sleeping pills. Sleeping-pill consumption increases with age and education.

8. People around the world spent $58 billion on sleep-aid products in 2014.

9. The most common sleep pharmaceutical drug is zolpidem, which you probably know as Ambien and is sold under other names. In 2013 the FDA cut the recommended dose of zolpidem in half.

10. Caffeine hinders our ability to fall asleep at night. After 2 P.M. is roughly the time sleep experts recommend we stop consuming caffeinated drinks.

11. The Greeks and the Romans each had their gods of sleep: Hypnos for the Greeks, Somnus for the Romans.

12. Thomas Edison bragged that he never needed more than four or five hours a night.

13. When Napoleon was asked how much sleep is good, it is said he replied, "Six for a man, seven for a woman, eight for a fool."

14. In 1903, the first sleeping pill, barbital, sold under the brand name Veronal, was developed.

15. There is awareness that sleep helps us to perform better both physically and cognitively, to learn faster and generally, to be healthier.

16. Sleep involves a range of complex; functions associated with memory, our ability to learn, brain development and cleaning, appetite, immune function and aging.

17. Sleepwalking occurs in approximately 17% of children and 4% of adults.

18. Sleep deprivation results in higher levels of the stress hormone cortisol the next day.

19. One of the most important findings is that sleep is essentially like bringing in the overnight cleaning crew to clear the toxic waste proteins that accumulate between brain cells during the day.

20. Lack of sleep in older adults increases the pace of brain-ventricle enlargement and decreased cognitive performance.

21. Studies show that a decrease in the total amount of sleep can lower a man's testosterone.

22. Sleep deprivation puts us at greater risk of " succumbing to impulsive desires, poor attentional capacity, and compromised decision making.

23. In a trial of cognitive behavioral therapy versus taking temazepam, the sleep onset was reduced by 55% for cognitive behavioral therapy as opposed to 46.5% for those taking the sleep drug.

24. If your subconscious plays your dream a second time, pay attention to it.

25. A minimum of seven hours of sleep a night is essential for optimal health.

26.   A study in April 2015 in Norway found that toddlers who consistently slept less than ten hours a night developed more emotional and behavioral problems by age five.

27. Students who started school at 8:30 a.m. slept nearly an hour more and performed better on tests than those who began school at 7:30 a.m.

28. 94% of couples that slept with their bodies touching were "happy with their relationship."

29. Snoring happens when your airways narrow, resulting in a vibration of our throat's soft tissue as you breath. Suggestions to help- skip your evening nightcap, sleeping with a humidifier, and losing weight. Of course, there are always earplugs and noise-canceling headphones.

30. Ideal sleeping temperature is 60-66 degrees F. Sleep is disrupted when the temperature rises above 75 degrees or falls below 54 degrees.

31. Some of the food building blocks for sleep: foods that contain magnesium as nuts, leafy greens, B6 as fish beans, and tryptophan as chickpeas, seaweed or halibut. Other helpful foods are tart cherry juice, Brazil nuts, baked sweet potato, and whole grain crackers.

32. Avoid spicy foods and sugar products as ice cream at bedtime.

33.   One of the most popular herbs for sleep is lavender, which promotes healing and relaxation.

34. A sleep helping, breathing exercise is the 4-7-8 method rooted in the ancient Indian Practice of pranayama—inhale four counts, hold for seven counts and exhale through the mouth for eight counts.

35. Banish all tech devices from your bedroom at least 30 minutes before you turn off the lights.

36. Short naps prime our brains to function at a higher level. Data suggests a 30minute nap can reverse the hormonal impact of a night of poor sleep.

37. During a nap the right side of the brain, the side associated with creativity, is active, while the left side stays mostly quiet.

38. The body is super busy repairing muscle and tissues and replacing dead cells while we're sleeping, and for athletes that time is crucial. The more you train the more you should sleep.

17. YOUR MEDICAL MIND: How to Decide What is Right for You   by Jerome Groopman MD

Synopsis: A book helping one make various medical decisions by reviewing options and learning their effects.

1. People consider whether or not they should take medication or undergo a medical procedure.

2. Despite a rigorous education in medical school and residency training, we had never been taught how and why a patient might come to choose one treatment over another.

3. Doctors should listen carefully to the patient, because he is telling you the answer.

4. The first statin was discovered in 1972 by scientists in Japan. The drug worked by blocking an enzyme in the liver that makes cholesterol.

5. In 2006 the National Community Pharmacists Association found that 31% of people never filled their prescription and another 29% stopped taking the medication before the supply ran out.

6. Understanding statistics about the risks and benefits of a treatment is called "health literacy."

7. The United States Department of Health and Human Services has a web site where one can check your risk level of a heart attack by clicking on "Cholesterol."

8. Health literacy is broken down into three aspects: without treatment, knowing the positive or negative information, and understanding the risks of a therapy.

9. In 2009, some $5 billion was spent on drug ads, more than twice the total budget of the Food and Drug Administration.

10. One of the first skills that we learned as medical students was to "take a history" from a patient: consider family history, past medical history, and knowledge about others who suffered similar maladies.

11. Researchers tested a new anticancer treatment, cisplatinum, a drug based on the metal. When experimented on a patient, the man's cancer was completely gone three months later.

12. By taking one-half of the doctor's recommended dosage of a statin, in six weeks a patient's total cholesterol went from 238 to 160.

13. In 2002 the WHI found that the hormone replacement therapy for menopausal women did not prevent heart disease; in fact, it appeared to increase the risk of heart attack.

14. In our role as doctors, our aim is to help patients understand what makes sense for them, what treatments are right given their individual values and goals.

15. Graves' disease is a form of hyperthyroidism, an overactive thyroid gland.

16. There appears to be three treatments for Graves' disease: a radioactive iodine pill, medication that prevents the thyroid gland from making too much hormone or surgery to remove the gland. All three appear to be equally effective.

17. Patients should be aware that doctors and other experts may frame information in a way that reflects their own preferences.

18. The Farmingham Heart Study estimated that over a lifetime, atrial fibrillation or related rhythm called atrial flutter would occur in about 25% of the population.

19. Guidelines aren't engraved in stone; they are subjective and fully half were overturned at five and a half years.

20. When considering an important medical decision, patients are often advised to obtain a second opinion.

21. A rational choice would be a treatment that provides the highest expected utility. This would be the treatment that avoids the worst side effects and has the least negative impact on one's life.

22. Research studies show that all of us initially overestimate the impact of illness and its unpleasant side effects because we tend to focus on the negative and neglect the numerous positives in our lives.

23. When searching for a specialist, the most frequent referrals come from the patient's primary care physician.

24. Autonomy is a primary right of all patients.

18. AN AMERICAN SICKNESS by Elisabeth Rosenthal

Synopsis: How healthcare became big business from its simple start to its current complicated involvement of government, corporations and lobbyists.

1. American medical system has stopped focusing on health or even science. Now it's single-mindedly to its own profits.

2. The United States spends nearly 20% of its gross domestic product on healthcare-more than twice the average of developed countries.

3. The earliest health insurance policies were designed primarily to compensate for income lost while workers were ill.

4. The original Blue Cross Plans, then not-for- profit, were set up not to make money but to protect patient's savings and keep hospitals afloat.

5. Between 1940 and 1955, the number of Americans with health insurance skyrocketed from 10% to over 60%.

6. In 1993, before Blue Cross went for-profit, insurers spent 95 cents of every dollar of premiums on medical care. Now it is a lot less due to marketing, lobbying, administration and paying out or dividends. Medicare uses 98% of its funding for healthcare and only 2% for administration.

7. From 1997 to 2012, the cost of hospital services grew 149%, while the cost of physician services grew 55%.

8. In the late 1900's Providence Hospitals no longer wanted to pay a salary to doctors in the ER and clinics; instead, it would treat them as independent contractors. This turned them into a business.

9. In the 1980's head nurses were changed to clinical nurses-managers who were more adapt at the business of medicine.

10. There is no such thing as a fixed priced for a procedure or test. The uninsured pay the highest prices of all.

11. Congress passed a law in 1974 requiring state health-planning agencies to grant approval of need before hospitals could build new facilities or indulge in the purchase of expensive technology. In 1987 the low was rescinded.

12. Deloitte is ranked number one by revenue in all areas of healthcare consulting.

13. New machines were purchased based not on medical necessity or even utility but according to financial calculations.

14. Before the 1940's hospitals paid trainee stipends by building their costs into patient's charges. After World War II, the GI Bill subsidized training and then the creation of Medicare, in 1965, established this funding which amounts to about $15 billion a year.

15. Twenty-five years ago, rooms with four beds were common. Private rooms were rare.

16. In 1986 a statute called the Emergency Medical Treatment and Labor Act was designed to force hospitals not to turn away sick patients as pregnant women who were poor. However, this did not apply to physicians.

17. In 1906 Congress passed the Wiley Act (also known as the Pure Food and Drug Act), to monitor and regulate drug safety. It was replaced in 1938 by the Food, Drug, and Cosmetic Act.

18. The FDA yardstick for approval did not include any consideration of price or measure of cost-effectiveness- a metric that all other countries use.

19. The Bayh-Dole Act of 1980 permitted scientists, universities, and companies to obtain patents on products that evolved from research funded by the government.

20. Up until the 1980's drugs were cheap. Direct to user advertising rose to $4.2 billion in 2005 and by 2006 it made up nearly 40% of total pharmaceutical promotional spending. The Supreme Court protected drug advertising under the guise of free speech. New Zealand is the only other country to allow this.

21. With the removal of CFC propellants the usual price of the most common inhaled asthma medicine, albuterol, rose from about $10 to over $100. It costs $7 to $9 in Australia.

22. The number of pay-for-delay arrangements had increased since 2010 and resulted in no generic drug competition to produce cheaper alternatives.

23. Postoperative nausea and vomiting was $149 for Zofran, compared with $3 for droperidol, which studies showed worked equally well.

24. A promising new noninvasive stool test for colon cancer, called Cologuard, is now on the market. You can imagine how the colonoscopy industry is fighting acceptance.

25. In 1976 amendments to the 1938 Food, Drug, and Cosmetic Act defined three classes of devices that needed various levels of approval. The third level is the one which required far more testing and red tape than the other two levels. So device makers try to get their device in level 1 or 2.

26. From 2005 to 2009, 70% of the high-risk-device recalls involved products that had gone to market through the 510(k) class 2 and should have been in class 3.

27. In 1966 half of ambulance calls in the United States were still handled by morticians.

28. The Medicare Prescription Drug Act, signed by President George W. Bush on December 8, 2003 was the first prescription drug coverage for seniors.

29. The rest of the world since 1992 has used international disease codes but not the United States. It too until 2015 for U.S/ to employ the system because the medical billing system were figuring out how to game the system.

30. Dr. Faustman discovered a vaccine to reverse type 1 diabetes in genetically predisposed mice. However, she could not get funding for the human testing due to manufacturers concern that there would be no deed for their products in this lucrative market.

31. The medical industry spends nearly half a billion dollars each year and is the largest lobbying force in the country. The oil and gas industry spend about $130 million.

32. The major effect of health care consolidation was simply a huge rise in prices, economic research has now shown, because hospital conglomerates that have driven out competition can raise prices with abandon.

33. The first step under President Obama's HITECH Act was to require doctors and hospitals to go electronic with their record keeping.

34. By 2014, 52% percent of overdue debt on credit reports was due to medical bills and effecting their ability to get a mortgage or buy a car.

35. The ACS barred insurers from denying insurance or treatment to people with preexisting conditions and banned lifetime limits on insurance payouts.

36. Once all seniors were guaranteed drug coverage and were paying only a co-payment, drug companies raised prices-a lot. Insurers then responded by charging higher-percentage co-payments to discourage use.

37. Under the ACA, the percentage of uninsured Americans dropped from 18% in2013 to 11.9% in 2016. But still 20 million people without insurance.

38. Drug spending is only 10% and payments to doctors in only 20% of the health budget.

39. Medical debt is the single biggest cause of bankruptcy in the United States.

40. Other developed countries delivers healthcare for a fraction of what it costs here in the U.S. Countries as Germany and Japan set national fee schedules for some combination of medial encounters or supplies and medicines.

41. In the U.S. doctors now spend 1/6 of their time on administration and medical practices to hire extra staff to wrangle with insurers.

42. Canada, Australia and others use a Single Payer system that cuts private insurers out of most basic medical financial transactions.

43. The high cost of malpractice insurance and lawsuits is not a primary cause of expensive medicine in the U.S.

44. Some studies have shown that between 50 and 90% of hospital bills contain mistakes.

45. The healthcare industry spends $15 billion a year on advertising about the same as auto manufacturers.

46. The FDA would not prosecute individuals who ordered drugs for personal use for less than ninety days.

19. DOPESICK by Beth Macy
DEARLERS, DOCTORS, and THE DRUG COMPANY THAT ADDICTED AMERICA

Synopsis: How the opioid drug problem started in the United States and how the laws and drug programs effected the addicted. Included are many personal stories of addicted individuals in the system.

1. Drug overdose had taken the lives of 300,000 Americans over the past 15 years. It has killed more people than guns or car accidents, at a rate higher than the HIV epidemic at its peak.

2. The Opioid pill addiction first took root in the mid-1990s in Appalachia's area of coal miners, loggers, furniture makers, and their kids.

3. The FDA approved the drug OxyContin in 1995 for the Purdue Company in Stamford, Connecticut.

4. The state of withdrawal from this new drug was the same as the opium-addicted in China who had long referred it to as "yen." (What the modern-day addicted users called dopestick).

5. By the 1870s, injecting morphine was so popular among the upper classes in Europe and the United States that doctors used it for a variety of ailments. In the early 1890's you could buy heroin at any American drugstore. By 1924 the manufacture of heroin was outlawed, 26 years after Bayer's pill came to market.

6. The 1996 introduction of OxyContin coincided with the moment in medical history when doctors, hospitals, and accreditation boards were adopting the notion of pain as "the fifth vital sign."

7. Industrywide, pharmaceutical companies spent $4.04 billion in direct marketing to doctors in 2000, up 64% from 1996.

8. Jobs in coal mining, once the number-one industry in central Appalachia, were cut in half between 1983 and 2012 due to pollution regulations and competition from natural gas. Peddling pills was now the modern-day moonshining.

9. Opioid addiction is a lifelong and typically relapse filled disease, but remission can take as long as ten or more years.

10. In the early 1990s, probably ninety percent of the heroin market was still in cities like New York, Chicago, and Detroit.

11. The FDA regulators and Big Pharma executives had been holding private meetings since 2002, through a drug-industry-funded nonprofit.

12. To help burnish the law suits in the face of many legal, financial, and public-relation problems, Purdue Pharma, the manufacturer of OxyContin, hired former New York mayor and Republican insider Rudy Giuliani and his consulting firm.

13. The U. S. attorney in Maine had challenged Purdue Pharma's promotional techniques, with some success. He left his post in 2001 and joined Purdue Pharma.

14. The addiction rate among those prescribed opioids for chronic nonmalignant pain was as high as 56% in 1980.

15. Once a person becomes addicted, he loses his power of choice; his free will becomes hijacked along with the opioid receptors in his brain.

16. By 2016, for every unemployed American man between the ages of 22 and 55, an additional three were neither working nor looking for work. Disability claims nearly doubled from 1996 to 2015.

17. Some risk factors for addiction include poverty, unemployment, multigenerational trauma, and access to drugs.

18. The highest per capita rate of heroin use in the country was Baltimore.

19. Americans, represent 4.4 % of the world's population and consume roughly 30% of its opioids.

20. In October 2014, hydrocodine-based painkillers such as Vicodin and Lortab were changed from Schedule III drugs to Schedule II, the same category as OxyContin.

21. With the legalization of marijuana in a growing number of states, drug cartels were champing at the bit to meet the demand for heroin.

22. Medicaid expansion was passed became the most important epidemic-fighting tool, paying for treatment, counseling and addiction medication.

23. The birth of methadone, a synthetic painkiller, developed for battlefield injuries was recovered from German labs shortly after World War II. American researchers learned that methadone quelled opioid withdrawal symptom but the Federal Bureau of Narcotics was against using drugs to treat drug addiction.

24. The Baltimore the needle-exchange initiative is credited with reducing needle-injected HIV instances from 64% to 8%.

25. The get tough-on-crime narrative fostered the shift in public spending from health and welfare programs to a massive system of incarceration. Imprisonment and correction spending went from $6.9 billion in 1980 to $80 billion today.

26. In the 1970's, America decided to deal with drug addiction and dependence as a crime problem rather than a health problem. Portugal, which decriminalized all drugs, including cocaine and

heroin, in 2001, and adding housing, food, and job assistance, now has the lowest drug-use rate in the European Union.

27. Painkillers aren't tobacco. Opioids have legitimate medical benefits when prescribed and used correctly.

28. People with addiction require help to get off of drugs, rather than simply treating them as criminals who have no right to health care.

29. Donald Trump performed best in the 2016 election in the most economic distress and the highest rates of drug, alcohol, and suicide mortality.

30. The explosive costs of addiction-related illness will eventually force health systems to integrate addiction treatment into general health care.

31. Instead of putting drug users in jail with its explosive jail cost and private prison expansion, we should be treating drug use as a disease and require treating them. The government had a program that paid Police departments for every drug user they arrested and jailed.

20. ADHA DOES NOT EXIST by Richard Saul, M.D.
The truth about attention deficit and hyperactivity disorder

Synopsis: A review of ADHD and the many ways that it could be misdiagnosed while offering some suggestions on the treatment of its cause.

1. Diagnosing and treating both children and adults has helped confirm my view that attention deficit and hyperactivity are primarily symptoms of other conditions.

2. There are many reasons for the misdiagnosis of ADHD, driven by patients, physicians, pharmaceutical companies and the media.

3. Over 4% of all adults and 11% of U.S. children are diagnosed with ADHD.

4. Harvard University research released in 2013 that some of the same genetic patterns underlie autism, depression, bipolar disorder, schizophrenia and ADHA.

5. Prescriptions for stimulants like Ritalin and Adderall are often prescribed for the wrong reasons as to improve test scores and professionals pulling long hours at the office.

6. Problems related to vision are among the most overlooked explanations for ADHA symptoms.

7. About 40% of all people are nearsighted, with the condition first appearing in childhood and peaking by early adulthood.

8. Symptoms of sleep disturbance, including poor concentration, and distractibility, may be mistaken for ADHD.

9. Seven hours is the well-documented minimum amount of sleep required for adults to avoid attention related and other cognitive deficits.

10. Chronic substance abuse, or the recurrent overuse of legal or illicit drugs or alcohol, is likely to result in distractibility and attention deficits that can be mistaken for ADHD.

11. The two main forms of substance-abuse treatment are medication and counseling.

12. The main clue to a possible bipolar disorder diagnosis is the presence of alternating periods of energetic, "up" moods and depression. At times misdiagnosed as ASHS.

13. Bipolar disorder is usually treated with a combination of medication and psychotherapy.

14. Difficulty with hearing is a surprisingly common source of attention-deficit/hyperactivity symptoms, especially in children.

15. About 17% of all U.S. adults report at least some degree of hearing loss- men more likely than women.

16. Some who struggle with a learning disability such as dyslexia may exhibit context-specific poor focus, and fidgeting that can be mistaken for ADHS.

17. Sensory processing disorder (SPD) involves difficulty integrating and organizing multiple types of signals to develop the most appropriate response in a range of everyday situations-from eating to playing a sport. There is no specific cure for SPD but the general approach known as occupational therapy, or helping patients improve their ability to carry out activities of daily living.

18. Gifted individuals can easily become bored and inattentive which could be misdiagnosed as ADHD. A treatment would be to give them increasing level of challenge in areas where they display more talent.

19. Hard –to-detect seizure disorders often exhibit short attention spans and distractibility that may be mistaken for ADHD. A seizure is

sometimes described as an electrical storm in the brain leading to abnormal movements. Increasing medication can actually increase the frequency of seizures. This applies to about 4% of the population.

20. There are about 20 drugs approved for treatment of epilepsy in the United States. Most fall into a category known as "anticonvulsants."

21. OCD (obsessive-compulsive disorder) is a mental disorder marked by obsessive thoughts and compulsive behavior aimed mostly at reducing obsessions. This sometimes is misdiagnosed as ADHD. About 2.5% of the population will be diagnosed with OCD at some point in their lives and a treatment- might consist of medication and psychotherapy.

22. Childhood fidgeting, distractibility, and impulsivity are often viewed as signs of ADHS. It could be better explained by Tourette's syndrome, a condition involving significant motor and vocal tics.

23. Asperger Syndrome, a difficulty paying attention, (an autism spectrum disorder) can be mistaken as ADHD

24. Sometimes ADHD symptoms can result from abnormal levels of the neurotransmitters serotonin and epinephrine/norepinephrine in the nervous system. The only way to confirm the condition is through blood tests.

25. Schizophrenia is a disorder that can occur in children and adults, and is marked by visual and auditory hallucinations, delusional beliefs, and can be mistaken for ADHD. When misdiagnosed as ADHD, patients are likely to be treated with stimulants, which fail to alleviate the symptoms and may even make them worse.

26. Fetal Alcohol Syndrome (caused by drinking during pregnancy) has a lifelong effect on a child including developmental and learning delays along with some physical characteristics and behavioral symptoms. The child could be wrongly diagnosed as ADHD. Help includes physical and occupational therapy.

27. Some symptoms that could result in misdiagnosis of ADHS: poor diet, allergies, overactive thyroid, prematurity and heavy metal poisoning.

28. A good starting point for anyone dealing with medical/behavioral symptoms is with some simple questions as: 1. What are your biggest

problems, 2. What are your strengths and weaknesses, 3. What do you think other people see as being your problems.
29. Some suggestions to patients: improve one's diet, exercise more, reduce harmful habits like smoking and illicit drug use, sleep more, and practice your passion.

21. HALLUCINATIONS by Oliver Sacks
Synopsis: An in-depth review of various types of hallucinations and their possible causes.

1. Generally, hallucinations are defined as percepts arising in the absence of any external reality- seeing things or hearing things that are not there.
2. Charles Bonnet syndrome was considered a hallucination of the brain to the loss of eyesight or other ocular problems. An activity drawing on memory now that it could no longer draw on sensation.
3. By far the commonest hallucinations are the geometrical ones: squares, checkerboards, tiles, walls, etc.
6. When there are colored hallucinations, there are activation of areas in the visual cortex associated with color construction. When there are auditory hallucinations, they may be associated with abnormal activation of the primary auditory cortex.
7. No one can have hallucinations of musical notation or numbers or letters if they have not actually seen these at some point in real life.
8. Hallucinations are marked by a lack of interaction. They are always silent and neutral. They rarely convey or evoke any emotion.
9. Sleep and dream deprivation beyond a few days may lead to hallucination. This can also occur from unprecedented experiences when the brain is released from the constraints of reality.
10. Until the eighteenth century, voices-like visions- were ascribed to supernatural agencies like gods or demons. They were simply accepted a part of human nature.
11. Hallucinations may arise from a stroke, a tumor, an aneurysm, an infectious disease, a neurodegenerative process, or toxic or metabolic disturbances.

12. Some people have musical hallucinations virtually nonstop, while others have them only intermittently. Music calls upon many areas of the brain.

13. Virtually everyone diagnosed with Parkinson's was medicated with L-dopa or other drugs that enhance the neurotransmitter dopamine in the brain. Hallucinations may occur months or years after taking these drugs.

14. Damage in parts of the brain stem, the midbrain and the pons causing lesions in the visual pathway could cause hallucinations.

15. In the 1950's when LSD, psilocybin mushrooms and morning glory seeds became widely available, ushered in the wave of hallucinogenic drug age and a new word-"psychedelic."

16. Sudden accelerations, slowing, or freezing of movement are also common with more elementary hallucinatory patterns.

17. Epileptic attacks are based on abnormal electrical discharge in the brain. This discharge arises from both halves of the brain simultaneously and can cause hallucinations.

18. Impairment or loss of vision to one side may lead to hallucinations in the blind or purblind area. Hallucinations may appear almost immediately with sudden damage to the occipital cortex of the brain.

19. Delirium caused by infections with high fevers or by problems like liver or kidney failure among others, and medications risk the increases of hallucinations.

20. Fevers are perhaps the commonest cause of delirium.

21. Activation of a homologous area in the left hemisphere may produce lexical hallucinations- of letters, numbers, musical notation, etc.

22. The central contrasts between sleep-related hallucinations and dreaming is that sleep-related are apt to be remembered in great detail.

23. Damage to the hypothalamus, from a head injury or tumor or disease, can cause narcolepsy later in life, which may cause hallucinations.

24. Most people enter the REM (rapid eye movement) stage ninety minutes or so after falling asleep, but people with narcolepsy may fall into REM at the very onset of sleep and wake at the wrong time and with visions persisting into the waking state.

25. The "mare" in "nightmare" originally referred to a demonic woman who suffocated sleepers by lying on their chests (she was called "Old Hag" in Newfoundland).

26. Any consuming passion, threat, loss or grief may lead to hallucinations in which an idea and an intense emotion are embedded.

27. Soldiers who had lost limbs in the Civil War, were the first to understand the neurological nature of phantom limbs. These phantom limbs are hallucinations in perceptions, but not quite comparable to hallucination of sight and sound.

22. SUCCESSFUL AGING by Daniel J. Levitin
   A Neuroscientist Explores the Power and Potential of
   Our Lives

Synopsis: A review and some helpful items to explore while we age. Included are functions of the brain, medications, sleeping and eating habits, and other items to help us along our journey of life.

1. Older minds might process formation more slowly than younger ones, but they can intuitively synthesize a lifetime of information and make smarter decisions based on decades of learning.

2. Our bodies react to insults, both psychological and physical, by releasing cortisol, the stress hormone. This reduces immune-system function, libido, and digestion.

3. Sleep deprivation in the aged is directly responsible for cognitive decline.

4. A good lifestyle concept (COACH) has five parts: Curiosity, Openness, Associations, Conscientiousness, and Healthy practices.

5. Successful aging has three aims: first- harness our knowledge so that we can anticipate changes, second-think about what ingredients presage a feeling of life well-lived when we look back from the end of life, and third-looking at the science of the brain and its aging process.

6. Five dimensions of personality: extraversion, agreeableness, conscientiousness, emotional stability and openness to experience.

7. Older adults are generally more concerned with making a good impression, and with cooperating and getting along with others.

8. Stress reduction is one of the most important things you can do for your overall health.

9. The key to remembering things is to get involved in them actively. Passively learning something, such as listening in a lecture, is a sure way to forget it. It helps to write things down and make a list that you want to remember.

10. Humans have 99% of our DNA in common with chimps. A banana has 60% in common with our DNA.

11. Sign language can be learned early by deaf children in the same way a child learns a language.

12. Dopamine levels fall about 10% per decade, and serotonin- and brain-derived neurotrophic factor levels also fall off with increasing age.

13. Cognitive reserve is the idea that people with more education and who are more intelligent may be able to withstand biological degradation better than others.

14. Dementia is a catchall term used to describe any brain disorder that causes deficits in more than one cognitive domain, such as attention, memory, and language.

15. Two of the most protective things you can do against aging is to keep up the manual skills learned when you were younger and start learning something new when you're old.

16. Starting at age sixty, you should have your eyes examined every two years.

17. The loss of flavor can result from normal age-related declines in the sensory receptors themselves, but in many cases, they result from diseases or medications.

18. Aging is not accompanied by unavoidable cognitive decline. The aging brain changes itself, heals itself, and finds other ways to do thigs. What helps is high levels of education and a balanced diet.

19. Some ways to reduce stress: exercise, meditation, listening to music, immersing yourself in nature, and sometimes just talking to friends and having social support.

20. Depression is an illness with biological causes and can often show up as lethargy, lack of motivation, and lack of energy, rather than

sadness. Some prescription medications have been associated with depression as estrogen, blood pressure medication, statins, and opioids.

21.   Three factors that have protected older individuals from depression are: 1. Presence of resources, 2. Psychological resources, and 3. Meaningful engagement with other people through social activities.

22. One of the surest ways to get over depression is to help others- this allows you to step outside of yourself and limit your preoccupations.

23. A feature of aging is that both sex-linked hormones, testosterone and estrogen, decline with age and these declines have well-documented effects.

24. Immersing yourself fully in whatever activities you engage in - work leisure, family, community- are protective against cognitive decline and physical illness.

25. Two knowledge domains that are most important to older adults are personal health and finance, and acquiring new information about each.

26. One of the keys to a long health span and a long life is social connectedness. Loneliness is associated with early mortality and the likelihood of developing Alzheimer's disease.

27.   Research suggests that religious people feel happier because religion promotes gratitude through prayers and gives them a social network.

28. One of the most common features of old age is aches and pains. The brain is wired in such a way that cognition, emotion, and pain can all interact with one another bidirectionally.

29. Fifty percent of nonsteroidal anti-inflammatory agent (NSAID) prescriptions are for arthritis and is the most prevalent pain condition in the United States. Although helpful, gels and creams are meant only to be absorbed by the skin and after an hour or two there is no more to be absorbed.

30. Untreated, chronic pain disrupts sleep patterns, which in turn can cause profound defects in memory and mood.

31. After age 70 it is suggested to make important decisions, those about finances, health, and the like, before noon. Your thinking is normally better in the morning.

32. Sleep hygiene involves avoiding bright lights before bed, sleeping in a dark room, and going to bed and waking at the same time every day.

33. About your diet: eating within two hours of bedtime can decouple the internal time rhythms. Alcohol and caffeine is known to disrupt sleep cycles, and high fat diets tend to advance your internal clock.

34. Terms like purify, detoxify, and energize are generally used to cover up a lack of scientific proof.

35. Insoluble fibers such as wheat bran, vegetables, and whole grains are healthy because they help prevent constipation and diverticulitis. It also appears that eating less helps longevity.

36. Foods related to health and against many forms of cancer include: brussels sprouts, broccoli, cauliflower, kale, cabbage and bok choy.

37. Constipation is one of the most common and annoying problems of aging, affecting 50% of older adults. It is treated by increasing consumption of insoluble fibers, such as bran, whole grains, vegetables, fluids and exercise.

38. Active engagement with the environment, as gardening, is helpful but when lost, it affects cognition through- dexterity, motivation, and loss of joy and pleasure at doing things for oneself.

39. Sleep deprivation is associated with Alzheimer's. When you're sleep-deprived those brain amyloid deposits don't get cleaned out, which keeps the brain functioning properly.

40. Naps can compensate for poor nighttime sleep, but it's best to limit them to twenty minutes or you can suffer from sleep inertia- your body wanting to stay asleep longer.

41. There is no convincing evidence that brain-training games enhance cognition beyond the realm of the game, nor do they fend off dementia.

42. Vitamin B12 deficiency is associated with cognitive decline. A study has shown that individuals who consumed more than two portions of mushrooms a week reduced their odds of having mild cognitive impairment by 50%.

43. Meditation is not going to cure your disease but it can help to make your brain more effective and more efficient.

44. Couples who are more satisfied with their spouses have increased longevity- up to 25%.

45. Some helpful hints for those who are developing Alzheimer's and mild cognitive impairment: 1. write your address on your cell phone and a card in your wallet which includes phone number and names of your doctor, spouse, and a family member or friend, 2. Start using pill-sorting box for your medications, 3. Keep your keys and wallet in a designated place. 4. Draw up an Advance medical directive and living will.

23. UNACCOUTABLE   by Marty Makary, MD
What hospitals won't tell you and how transparency can revolutionize health care

Synopsis: A review of the inner activities in hospitals and the activities of doctors that effect the patient and medical cost.

1. New England Journal of Medicine reported that as many as 25% of all patients are harmed by medical mistakes.

2. Drug companies and device manufacturers sometimes give large kickbacks to doctors, which is rarely disclosed to patients.

3. Studies revealed that teamwork culture could vary dramatically within a hospital. All depending on the culture of the hierarchy.

4. Although it is not mandatory for hospitals to publicly report safety-survey results, there is a free version of it on the Department of Health and Human Services' website: www.ahrq.gov/qual/patientsafetyculture.

5. Two trends in modern medicine: 1) hospital administration being removed from daily hospital care, and 2) modern medicine's growing appetite to overscreen, overdiagnoses, and overtreat.

6. Only one third of heart centers have voluntarily allowed their outcomes to be posted on the STS (The Society of Thoracic Surgeons) website.

7. New York State's public reporting experiment in heart surgery showed that high-volume doctors performed much better than low-volume doctors. "Practice makes Perfect."

8. When choosing a hospital, beware of clever marketing. Insist on finding out how many patients they treat each year for your condition.

9. Ask the right questions about your condition such as: Are there other ways of treat this? What % of these operations are done open versus a minimally invasive way? How many days will I be in the hospital with this operation? and Get a second opinion.

10. In the right hands, minimally invasive surgery is safer and has numerous benefits, many of which are heralded as the future of health care.

11. Benefits of minimally invasive surgery: less pain, fewer infections, shorter hospitalization, lower medication use during recovery and earlier return to work.

12. The laparoscopic revolution in America was a non-university hospital phenomenon that began in community hospitals.

13. The two types of doctors required by the average person are proceduralists who do the operation or set the procedures and the diagnosticians who figure out what is wrong.

14. When further testing is recommended, be sure to ask what the incremental benefit is, since it can sometimes be avoided.

15. Rates of serious substance abuse and psychiatric disease among doctors are actually higher than that of other professions with similar educational background and socioeconomic status.

16. William Halsted, considered by many to be the father of American surgery, is credited with the first radical mastectomy for breast cancer and the introduction of surgical gloves- before that, doctors operated with bare hands.

17. A 2009 study from the Archives of Internal Medicine found that 31% of doctors get burned out and 51% of doctors wouldn't recommend the profession to one of their children.

18. Hospitals find it is cheaper to settle claims out of court. In fact, hospital lawyers go to court on average only once for every ten to twenty lawsuits.

19. The more revenue a doctor brings in, the weaker the hospital's incentive to look into local allegations against him.

20. A 2011 report found that a small fraction of doctors disciplined by their hospital are often not reported to their state medical board.

21. A New England Journal of Medicine study concluded that as many as 25% of all hospitalized patients will experience a preventable medical error of some kind.

22. When a doctor or hospital does harm to a patient, the settlement offer from the hospital often contains a confidentiality clause (a gag rule).

23. Medical mistakes are a heavy tax on our society via costs that are passed on in the form of higher medical bills, higher insurance premiums, and higher deductibles.

24. If giving to a children's hospital pick a local nonprofit who will show you exactly how your money will be used to help children, and what your money will be used to buy. Remember tax-free children's hospitals make record profits and pay their executives record salaries.

25. Only one quarter of pancreas cancers respond to chemo, and patients who do chemo live only about one month longer on average. A trial in European cooperative group showed no benefit to radiation. Yet radiation is common treatment in the United States.

26. Whenever confronted with a medical decision, inquire about the difference in average outcomes and quality of life among the options.

27. Recent disclosure rules are requiring that doctors report money received from drug and device companies, but the disclosure is not shared with the patient.

28. In the 2011 Journal of the American Medical Association study that one in five patients who received heart defibrillators didn't meet guidelines to have them placed.

29. Recently concluded study concluded from a comprehensive analysis of America's ten-year experience with robotic surgery that there is not strong evidence to support a benefit to patients. It is mainly a marketing hook to attract patients.

30. The U.S. now owns four times as many surgeon robots as all other countries in the world combined.

31. In a recent study, nurses rated their teamwork and communication with doctors as bad (48%), contradicting doctors reported as great (85%).
32. Checklists and medical-unit group meetings with administrators are a few common-sense solutions that are quickly gaining attention in health care.
33. The complication rates a doctor will quote out of text books and the medical literature, however, are generally two to three times higher in the real world.
34. Modern medicine's general lack of accountability is a problem that doesn't just annoy patients but bothers many doctors who are at the top of their field.
35. When operation videos were to time and score procedures, all of a sudden, the average length of the procedures done by doctors increased by 50% and the quality score increased by 30%.
36. Making operation video records available to patients and their doctors is a game changer and can strengthen the patient-doctor trust.
37. The average American has 9.2 procedures in a lifetime, according to a study by Dr. Atul Gawande.
38. Hospitals are not required to report their complication rates, readmission rates, or other standardized metrics of how they are performing.
39. Nurses play a central role as mediators between patients and the rest of the hospital system. Their organization has campaigned to encourage nurses to speak up when something doesn't look right.
40. The Institute for Healthcare Improvement, a national resource center created to help hospitals perform better, focus on reducing error rates and implementing best practices

24. SUPER BRAIN by Deepak Chopra, M.D. and Rudolph E. Tanzi, Ph.D.

Unleashing the explosive power or your mind to maximize health, happiness, and spiritual well being

Synopsis: An in-depth view of the mind and brain with some technical input, and how it affects us and how we can affect it.

1. Your brain contains roughly 100 billion nerve cells forming anywhere from a trillion to perhaps even a quadrillion connection called synapses.
2. Super brain stands for a fully aware creator using the brain to maximum advantage. Your brain is endlessly adaptable, and you could be performing a fourfold role- leader, inventor, teacher, and user.
3. We now know that babies are born with 90 percent of their brains formed. So the first years of life are spent winnowing out the unused connections and growing the ones that will lead to new skills.
4. By setting higher expectations, you enter a phase of higher functioning. One of the unique things about the human brain is that it can do only what it thinks it can do.
5. The vagus nerve runs to the brain along the carotid artery in the throat, and it is involved in regulating some major functions- heart rate, sweating, muscle movements for speech and keeping the larynx open for breathing.
6. As the saying goes, you don't know you have Alzheimer's because you forget where you put your car keys. You know you have Alzheimer's when you forget what they are for.
7. The human brain loses about one cortical neuron per second. But this is an infinitesimal fraction of the roughly 40 billion neurons in your cerebral cortex.
8. By choosing to exercise every day, you can increase the number of new nerve cells, just as you do when you actively seek to learn new things.
9. Phobias can be successfully treated by bringing in awareness and restoring control to the user of the brain where it belongs.
10. Every time you complain "My memory is going," you reinforce that message in your brain. What you should be looking at is habit, behavior, attention, enthusiasm, and focus, all of which are primarily mental.

11. If you are getting older and feel that memory loss could be occurring, focus your effort on mental activity that besets brain function.

12. Being a fully integrated person means having three strengths that reflect a baby's approach to the world and avoiding three obstacles that plague us as adults: Strengths- communicating, staying balanced, seeing the big picture; obstacles- isolation, conflict, repression.

13. Buddha is more than Buddhism. The greatest spiritual guides exemplify three strengths and avoid three obstacles: Strengths- evolving, expanding, being inspired: obstacles- contraction, fixed boundaries, conformity.

14. Heroes of super brain aren't the same as super heroes. They are realistic models for change. We believe that the continual development of super brain will lead to a healthier and more highly functioning brain.

15. Depression is classified as a mood disorder, traceable to the brain's inability to react properly to inner and outer stress. It affects the whole body. Once the brain has been triggered the first time, the brain changes. In the future it takes smaller and smaller triggers to enter depression, until finally almost none is needed.

16. The person who wants to avoid depression must first stop exposing yourself to stresses that occur over and over. It's important to deal with the problems more promptly and directly than you otherwise might.

17. The mind, brain, and body work seamlessly together. The deeper you master this process the closer you are to arriving at the goal of super brain.

18. Stress alleviating activities, such as doing physical exercise and learning new things promote the birth of new nerve cells, which promotes new synapses and neural circuits.

19. Every quality in the outside world exists because you create it. Your brain is not the creator but a translational tool. The real creator is mind.

20. Because brain tissue cannot feel physical pain, open-brain surgery can be performed with the patient awake.

21. It's good to be aware, but self-awareness is even better. Knowing where your anger comes from adds the component of self-awareness. It allows you to see a pattern in your behavior.

22. The brain is fluid and dynamic. When you constrict your awareness, you constrict the brain and freeze your reality into fixed patterns.

23. More than one-third of Americans are overweight. The key to getting it under control is to bring your brain into balance then use its ability to balance everything- hormones, hunger, cravings, and habits.

24. The brain has neither will nor intention; only the mind does. Mind isn't physical, but if you sweep mind aside, you can study the brain on purely physical grounds.

25. Too intense a desire for success leads to stronger fears of failure and if fear rises, it can create failure.

26. Medical studies have found only a few things that the mind-body system cannot adapt to: one of them is chronic pain, and the other is anxiety.

27. Fear and desire are bred in your instinctive brain, mediated by your emotional brain, and negotiated by your intellectual brain.

28. In humans, the intellectual phase of the brain blends instinctive drives and emotions with knowledge gained from experience.

29. Neuroscience has divided the mind into instinct, intellect, and emotions and has mapped the regions of the brain corresponding to each.

30. If you don't develop your intellect, it remains stuck in rudimentary thinking. You become the pawn of influences from outside yourself.

31. Highly successful people, when asked how they reached the top, tend to agree on two things: they were very lucky, and they would up in the right place at the right time.

32. As you grow older, your tendency is to narrow your likes and dislikes, which means that you are denying your brain its ability to be holistic.

33. Sit down and write your personal vision. Aim for the highest goals you can imagine that would bring fulfillment.

34. A healthy brain is benefited from: 1. Inner works- sleep time, focus time, time in, down time, 2. Outer time- physical exercise, play time, connection time.

35. Your body knows at a subtle level where disease and discomfort are. It sends signals at every moment, and such signals are not to be feared.

36. The secret to compliance of weight control isn't exerting more willpower or beating yourself up for not being perfect. The secret is changing without force. Anything you force yourself to do will eventually fail.

37. Older people on average take seven prescribed medications, all of which have side effects. The focus on drugs has lessened the public incentive to practice prevention, which has no side effects and proven benefits.

38. A study by Sara Konrath of the University of Michigan found that individuals who volunteer lived longer than nonvolunteers.

39. Dying is a process that passes through stages. By now those stages are familiar: grief, denial, anger, bargaining, depression, and acceptance.

40. Super brain depends upon a growing self-awareness, so being mindful is crucial. Mindfulness can be cultivated through meditation. Sit in a quiet place, close your eyes, take deep breaths and let your body relax.

41. In the terminology of neuroscience, all the colors, sounds, and textures that we experience are lumped together under the term qualia. Regaining control over qualia is the key to reshaping the brain and your personal reality at the same time.

42. In the brain all experience must be processed through chemical pathways, much as the raw energy in food is metabolized.

43. Behavior shapes biology. Research has shown that positive lifestyle changes in diet, exercise, stress management and meditation affect our genes and the brain.

44. We must never forget that the rue set of human existence is in the mind, to which the brain bows like the most devoted and intimate of servants.

. 25. THE PATIENT SURVIVAL GUIDE
 by Dr. Maryanne McGuckin with Toni L. Goldfarb

Synopsis: Some interesting information to guide you on possible health problems that might occur and some hints to stay healthy.

1. One out of every 20 people develop an infection while they are in the hospital. These ae called "healthcare associated" infections.
2. Three ways to reduce your risk: 1. Ask all who enter your room to wash their hands, 2. You wash your hands after touching anything as toilet, food tray, etc., 3. Do not shake hands with anyone.
3. During the 1800's many women were dying after child birth due to dirty hands.
4. Bacteria are in three shapes: balls, rods, or spirals.
5. Viruses live inside your cells, where antibiotics can't get to them.
6. Any infection a patient develops 48 hours after hospital admission is considered to be healthcare associated.
7. There are four major categories of infections: urinary, respiratory, surgical, and bloodstream infections.
8. Hospitals are required to find out what causes any infection a patient develops, and they know how to do it.
9. You have a right to see the hospitals Joint Commission infection surveillance report.
10. The three most common super bugs: MRSA, VRE and C.diff
11. Medical gloves are meant for only one use and the wearer should immediately wash their hands after their use.
12. Hospital infection prevention checklist: 1. Ask the hospital's infection rates, 2. Demand a room without an infected patient, 3. Ask all workers to wash their hands.
13. If too weak to ask questions or pay-attention, get an advocate as a family member, a friend, or a paid professional. What you desire should be in a living will and given to the advocate.
14. Hospital consent forms can be long and in tiny print so have the hospital send you a copy to review well before your procedure.
15. Review and ask if the surgery is necessary and what are the alternatives?
16. Six things to know before you sign an Informed Consent Form: 1. Patient's Diagnosis, 2. Purpose of proposed treatment, 3. Risks of not

having the procedure, 4. benefits of the procedure, 5. Alternatives to treatment and, 6. Risks of the alternatives

17. Urinary infections are the most common healthcare-associated infections. The tract includes kidneys, ureters, bladder and urethra.

18. The pneumococcal pneumonia vaccine is generally recommended for people aged 65 years and older.

19. Overuse of antibiotics should always be avoided because of the risk that pneumonia bacteria may become resistant to antibiotic treatment.

20. Daily oral care helps to decrease plaque and bacterial growth in the oral cavity, so that bacterial colonies don't form and infection doesn't begin.

21. Safety procedures are required at each stage of an operation: pre-op, operative, post-op, and post-discharge.

22. Some of the personal factors that can increase your risk of infection after surgery: diabetes, cigarette smoking, use of steroids, being overweight.

23. Be alert for signs and symptoms of an infection: redness, swelling, heat, pain, drainage and odor.

24. Items to consider before leaving the hospital: instructions on care, home care activities, bathing, name and phone number of a healthcare representative for the hospital, schedule a follow-up appointment.

25. Guidelines of the CDC for healthcare workers to prevent bloodstream infections: sterile precautions during a catheter insertion, skin cleaning, and removal of catheters when no longer needed.

26. Two important things in this book: stay informed and empowered, wash your hands, and insist that healthcare workers do the same,

27. Pregnant women should check on hospital nurseries far in advance of their due date

28. Medicare regulations now require member centers to follow infection control guidelines.

29. Advice for every patient treated at ambulatory surgery facilities: be sure it is affiliated with a hospital, bring your list of medicines,

before leaving ask about potential complications, and get a list of prescriptions to fill and ask what each is for.

30. About 1 million people in the United States currently reside in assisted living facilities. That number is projected to double by 2030.

31. Assisted living facilities are not subject to federal government regulation. However, all 50 states license or certify these facilities.

32. Nursing homes are required by law to follow the same infection control guidelines that hospitals must follow.

33. If a malpractice is filed you will probably get no more that 50% of any money awarded due to legal and processing fees.

34. Three categories of recoverable damages in cases involving wrongful action that causes harm: a. tort action, b. compensatory, c. punitive and d. nominal.

26. Body Brokers by Annie Cheney
Inside America's Underground Trade in Human Remains.

Synopsis: A review and some history of what happens to body parts and how they are acquired for medical schools, research, and surgical operations.

1. Every year in the United States, tens of thousands of corpses enter the cadaver trade. Corpses that enter this business are cut up into parts and distributed through a complex network of suppliers, brokers, and buyers.

2. Each corpse that travels through the system can generate anywhere from $10,000 to $100,000, depending on how it is used.

3. Only ten percent of states in the U.S. inspect crematoria or require their workers to be certified. Roughly half of all states have no laws governing cremation at all.

4. Today, roughly 10,000 cadavers a year are used to introduce U.S. medical students to the miracles of anatomy.

5. Corpses in various states of decay are packaged in body bags then in coffin-shaped cardboard boxes used for cremation.

6. Buyers of body parts don't ask questions. The donor's names are considered confidential, so the buyers never see consent forms. They

get a list of ID numbers and a package of parts, and take the supplier's word for the rest.

7. It is thought that it is not possible to regulate this business. It would be an arduous task to try and regulate it. You're going to have lobbyists like J and J. These toolers don't want regulations.

8. ScienceCare Anatomical, an Arizona company body broker, opened in June 2000. Within two years the company was selling body parts to major surgical-equipment companies such as Arthrex and Smith & Nephew – big companies with a great need for corpses.

9. For decades, live pigs were the specimen of choice for educating surgeons. During the 1990s, as courses in surgery began to focus on minimally invasive technique human corpses were used . Unlike human corpses, pigs bleed.

10. Florida is the only state in the country that requires vendors to get approval from the state anatomy board before shipping in body parts. Most come in undetected. In 1995, there were just two requests.

11. Companies that market minimally invasive technology- like Zimmer and US Surgical have built their own institutes, where surgeons can attend courses showcasing the company's devices.

12. The more hands-on courses that are available, the more the demand for brokers of body parts.

13. Companies have developed tricks for preserving the flesh. Before freezing a corpse, they massage Vicks VapoRub into the skin. That way when the body defrosts, the odor is of Menthol, not old cheese.

14. In the early 1800's the only bodies that could be legally dissected were those of hanged murderers. There weren't enough murderers to go around and so the surgeons depended on gangs of so-called resurrectionists, to supply them with" subjects."

15. The word surgery comes from the Greek "cheirourgia", which means, literally, hand work. The Greeks learned surgery from the ancient Egyptians.

16. In the Middle Ages much of the medical knowledge advanced by the Greeks and then Romans was lost. Papal law prohibited human dissection.

17. The Renaissance brought a renewed interest in medicine and specifically in human anatomy. In the sixteenth century, the Papal

ban on dissection was finally lifted. However, there was no reliable form of anesthesia, no understanding of bacteria or infection.

18. By the late 1780's dissection courses were being held in Vienna, Paris , as well as in London.

19. Dr. Astley Cooper was a great innovator of his time in the early 1800's. He was the first surgeon to tie the carotid artery for an aneurysm and the first to amputate a leg at the hip.

20. In 1832, partly as a result of two murders, the British government passed the Anatomy Act, which was intended to put an end to the cadaver trade in England once and for all. The new law provided surgeons with the "unclaimed" bodies of the poor and friendless for dissection.

21. In the early days of body snatching in America, ghouls (grave robbers) limited their activities to local graveyards, since they traveled by horse and wagon and had to have enough time to bring the corpses back to the medical schools before sunrise before the body would start to decompose. Later, the advent of railroads allowed them to travel farther afield to collect corpses.

22. When the states made it a crime to steal bodies, the price of corpses rose, but the surgeons and medical students continued to buy from the ghouls.

23. In 1831 Massachusetts passed the Anatomy Act. That law designated unclaimed bodies for anatomical dissection. In 1947, Tennessee was the last state to pass such a law.

24. Beginning in the 1950s, medical schools began to accept body donations from the public. The first state to legalize body donation was California. What fueled the underground cadaver trade of today was the number of accredited medical schools in the United States that grew from 88 to 126.

25. Unlike most states, Pennsylvania prohibits the exportation of body parts. The law also required that anyone receiving a donated body have a license from the state.

26. The American Association of Clinical Anatomists was founded in 1982 due to the concern that anatomy was losing favor in medical schools.

27. Between 1998 and 2005, criminal investigations have been launched into four different medical schools. But as of this time only one medical school employee has been indicted or served jail time.

28. It's common for medical schools with a surplus of donated bodies to share them with other schools. But in some cases, schools with a surplus of corpses hire middlemen to broker the bodies for them .

29. As long as there was little state regulation, no federal oversight, and a market for body parts the incidents of profiteering and theft would continue to plague schools.

30. All bodies undisturbed after death decay in the same way. The rate of decay depends on variables as temperature, humidity, place and cause of death. By the third day, a green tinge has spread around the torso and down the thighs. Bacteria now devour the flesh. And soon there is nothing left but bones.

31. There is a twelve-hour time limit that a donor body can remain without refrigeration if its tissue is meant to be transplanted.

32. The practice of transplanting human tissue began in the late 1940's as an experiment. Several surgeons had reported success transplanting frozen bone.

33. Surgeons routinely used cadaver ligaments and tendons to treat sports injuries. They discovered they could use cadaver menisci to replace torn menisci in the living.

34. In 1993, The FDA issued an interim rule, which required tissue banks to screen donors for risk factors and to test their tissue for diseases such as HIV and hepatitis.

35. As the tissue business had grown lucrative, medical device companies have started to move in. It was a natural with their salespeople, and surgeons and hospital contacts.,

.

27. BREATH   by James Nestor
The new Science of a lost art

Synopsis: A study on how we breath and how proper breathing can help cure some minor health problems.

1. Forty percent of today's population suffers from chronic nasal obstruction, and around half of us are habitual mouth breathers.

2. Mammals grow noses to warm and purify the air, throats to guide air into lungs, and a network of sacs that would remove oxygen from the atmosphere and transfer it into the blood.

3. Even though the ancient people never flossed, brushed, or saw a dentist, they all had straight teeth. They had forward facial growth and large mouths creating larger nose airways. It is unlikely that they ever snored or had sleep apnea.

4. In colder climates, our noses would grow narrower and longer to more efficiently heat up air before it entered our lungs.

5. As humans developed speech, the larynx sank, opened up space in the back of the mouth and allowing a wider range of vocalizations and volumes.

6. Anders Olsson spent about 10 years researching the differences in performance between nasal breathers and mouth breathers. He became convinced that mouth breathing can put the body into a state of stress that can make us more quickly fatigued and sap athletic performance.

7. Simply training yourself to breathe through your nose could cut total exertion in half and offer huge gains in endurance.

8. Inhaling from the nose has the effect of forcing air against the flabby tissues at the back of the throat, making the airways wider and breathing easier.

9. Forty-five percent of adults snore occasionally. A quarter of the population snores constantly. No amount of snoring is natural.

10. The nose is crucial because it clears air, heats it, and moistens it for easier absorption.

11. A study, by Dr. Mark Burhenne, has shown that mouth breathing contributed to periodontal disease and bad breath, and was the number one cause of cavities, even more damaging than sugar. He suggested to apply mouth tape at night if you snore.

12. Nasal breathing alone can boost nitric oxide sixfold which is one of the reasons we can absorb about 18 percent more oxygen than by just breathing through the mouth.

13. In the 1980's, researchers with the Framingham Study discovered that the greatest indicator of life span wasn't genetics, diet or the amount of daily exercise but was lung capacity.

14. The lungs themselves will lose about 12 percent of capacity from the age of 30 to 50 and will continue declining even faster as we get older. Moderate exercise like walking or cycling has been shown to boost lung size by up to 15 percent.

15. The diaphragm located at the base of the lungs helps the heart when extended. Extending your breaths to 50 to 70 percent of the diaphragm's capacity will ease cardiovascular stress.

16. Track runners are encouraged to never hold their breath when positioned at the starting line at the beginning of a race, but to breathe deeply and calmly and always exhale at the sound of the starter pistol.

17. We have about 100 times more carbon dioxide in our body than oxygen and that most of us need even more of it.

18. The best way to prevent chronic health problems, improve athletic performance, and extend longevity was to focus on how we breath. To do this we'd need to learn how to inhale and exhale slowly.

19. For a healthy body, over breathing or inhaling pure oxygen would have no benefit, no effect on oxygen delivery to our tissues and organs.

20. The key to optimum breathing and health is to practice fewer inhales and exhales in a smaller volume.

21. When we breath slower we hold in more carbon dioxide causing our pH to lower and blood become more acidic, all better for the body and lungs.

22. It was the constant stress of chewing that was lacking from our diets. Ninety-five percent of the modern, processed diet is soft. Our ancient ancestors chewed for hours a day and their faces grew to be wide and strong, pronounced, and had straight with no decay teeth.

23. The earliest orthodontics devices weren't intended to straighten teeth, but to widen the mouth and open airways. Devices invented to fix crooked teeth caused by too-small mouths were making mouths smaller and breathing worse.

24. Breathing is more than just a biochemical or physical act. It affects heart rate, digestion, moods, and attitudes.

25. The deeper and more softly we breathe in, and the longer we exhale, the more slowly the heart beats and the calmer we become.

26. Blends of 30 percent carbon dioxide and 70 percent oxygen became a go-to treatment for anxiety, epilepsy, and even schizophrenia. For some unknown reason, in the 1950's that research ended and that treatment changed to pills.

27. The concept of "prana" (vital energy), an ancient theory of atoms, was first documented in India and China. Spicy foods contained large doses of prana, which is one of the reasons traditional Indian and Chinese diets are often hot.

28. Cancers develop and thrive in environments of low oxygen. Breathing slow, less, and through the nose balances the levels of respiratory gases in the body and sends the maximum amount of oxygen to the maximum number of tissues.

29. Feeding the body with more air than it needs is damaging for the lungs right down to the cellular level.

30. For peak efficiency, James Nestor advises that the perfect breath is: Breathe in for about 5.5 seconds, then exhale for 5.5 seconds. That's 5.5 breaths a minute for a total of about 5.5 liters of air.

31. Breathing therapy can't cure everything but can help some body conditions and even minimize doctor's visits and some medications.

28. THE OBESITY CODE   by Jason Jung, MD
Unlocking the secrets of weight loss

Synopsis: A review of some of the technical causes of obesity and some helpful hints on how to help prevent and alleviate the situation.

1. Obesity is defined in terms of a person's body mass index, calculated as a person's weight in kilograms divided by the square of their height in meters. A body mass index greater than 30 is defined as obese.

2. Calorie reduction had been prescribed for the last fifty years with startling ineffectiveness.

3. All foods can be divided into three different macronutrient groups: fat, protein and carbohydrates.

4. From 1976 to 1996 the average fat intake decreased from 45 percent of calories to 35 percent while grains and sugars increased.

The increase in obesity began exactly with the officially sanctioned move toward a low-fat, high-carbohydrate diet.

5. Childhood obesity is associated with a 200 percent to 400 percent increased risk of adult obesity.

6. The root cause of obesity is a hormonal imbalance with high blood insulin as its central feature.

7. The key assumptions in the calorie reduction theory of weight loss have all been proven false. All calories are not equally likely to cause weight gain. Caloric reduction doesn't cause lasting weight loss.

8. Weight loss triggers two important responses. First, total energy expenditure is immediately reduced. Second, hormonal hunger signals an effort to acquire more food.

9. Increasing exercise does not reduce obesity. The vast majority (95%) of calories are used for basal metabolism as diet, body temperature, organ function, etc.

10. Insulin is a key regulator of energy metabolism. It is one of the fundamental hormones that promote fat accumulation and storage. Insulin facilitates the uptake of glucose into cells for energy.

11. Under normal conditions, high insulin levels encourage sugar and fat storage. Low insulin levels encourage glycogen and fat burning.

12. Numerous studies, conducted mostly on diabetic patients, have already demonstrated the fact that increased insulin levels in the body causes weight gain.

13. Cortisol (prepares the body for action) and insulin (a storage hormone) both have similar weight gain effects.

14. Insulin resistance leads directly to higher insulin levels, and increased insulin levels are a major driver of obesity.

15. Population studies consistently link short sleep duration with excess weight.

16. Despite being full, we always have room for highly refined carbohydrates like cake and pie - but not proteins or fats. Highly refined carbs do not trigger the release of satiety hormones.

17. A systematic review of all the dietary trials showed that much of the benefits of a low-carbohydrate approach evaporated after one year.

18. High insulin levels cause weight gain. Food choices play a role in raising insulin levels. Another pathway that increases insulin

independent of diet is Insulin resistance. It leads to high insulin levels in the body and causes obesity.

19. In 1977, most people ate three times a day. By 2003, most people were eating five to six times a day, which included snack time in between meals.

20. The vast majority (73%) of children regularly eat sugary cereals for breakfast.   By contrast, only 12 percent regularly eat eggs at breakfast.

21. Excessively high insulin resistance is the disease known as type 2 diabetes. It leads to elevated blood sugars, which are a symptom of this disease.   Giving insulin for type 2 diabetes will worsen, not improve the disease.

22. Mississippi is the poorest state in the U.S. It also has the highest level of obesity, at 35.4 percent.

23. Large scale consumption of highly processed carbohydrates leads to obesity.

24. Probably your grandmother was right in losing weight and attacking the central problem of obesity. Cut down on sugars and starches, and stop snacking. These strategies attack the worst offenders of insulin secretion and resistance.

25. Fructose, a sugar found naturally in fruit, is metabolized only in the liver and does not circulate in the blood. Fructose does not appreciably change the blood glucose level.

26. Insulin is normally released when we eat. It directs some of the incoming glucose to be used as energy and some to be stored for later use. Glucose is stored as glycogen in the liver. Excess glucose is stored as fat

27. Cutting back on sugars and sweets has always been the first step in weight reduction in virtually all diets throughout history. Don't replace them with artificial sweeteners.

28. Diet sodas do not reduce the risk of obesity, metabolic syndrome, strokes or heart attacks. That is because it is insulin, not calories that ultimately drives obesity and metabolic syndrome.

29. Refining carbohydrates significantly increases the glycemic index by purifying and concentrating the carbohydrate. It means that it can be digested and absorbed very quickly and encourages overconsumption.

30. Food fiber is beneficial in treating obesity. It may help decrease food intake, slow down food's absorption in the stomach and small intestine, and then help it exit quickly through the large intestines. Fiber increases satiety, reduces hunger and decreases caloric intake.

31.   Fiber can protect against elevated insulin and help protect against type 2 diabetes.

32. The use of olive oil and apple cider vinegar as salad dressing is associated with lower risk of cardiovascular disease. Vinegar actually seems to exert a protective effect on the serum insulin response.

33. When given by mouth, many medicines are incompletely absorbed or partially deactivated by the liver before reaching the bloodstream. For this reason, intravenous delivery tends to be much more effective.

34. After five years of follow-up, findings showed that total meat, red meat, poultry and processed meats were all significantly associated with weight gain.

35. A ten-year study found that the highest intake of dairy is associated with the lowest incidence of obesity and type 2 diabetes. Also, large observation studies do not link dairy consumption to weight gain.

36. Cholesterol is a key building block in the membranes that surround all the cells in our body. If you reduce cholesterol in your diet, your body will simply make more.

37. Omega 3 fatty acids decrease thrombosis (blood clots) and are believed to protect against heart disease. It is found in flax seeds, walnuts, and oily fish such as sardines and salmon.

38. Polyunsaturated fats, like most vegetable oils, are less stable chemically than saturated fats. Because of this, they have a tendency to go rancid and have a short shelf life. The solution was to create artificial trans-fats with longer shelf life. .

39. In 1990, Dutch researchers noted that consuming trans fats increased LDL, the bad cholesterol. It was estimated that a 2 percent increase in trans-fat consumption would increase the risk of heart disease by a whopping 23 percent.

40. Findings throughout the decades were that monounsaturated fats (olive oil) were protective against a stroke.

41. There is no one single cause of obesity. It combines with carbohydrates, insulin resistance, sugar, and calories.

42. As for desserts, other than the sugary ones, eat fresh seasonal fruit, dark chocolate (without milk chocolate) with more than 70 percent cacao, or a plate of nuts and cheeses.

43. Some simple food rules to follow: eat cereals containing less than 4 grams of sugar per serving, Greek yogurts - not the commercial yogurts with high levels of sugar, oatmeal as whole oats and steel-cut oats. These are a good choice but not the instant oatmeal as it is processed and contains large amounts of added sugar. Also, eggs are a good source of lutein and zeaxanthin.

44. Coffee, even decaffeinated version, appears to protect against type 2 diabetes and a major source of antioxidants as is green tea.

45. Fasting leaves more blood for your brain. Fasting is the most efficient and consistent strategy to decrease insulin levels. All foods raise insulin; therefore, it is effective at times to reduce insulin by avoiding food.

29. PRINCIPLES OF TRDITIONAL CHINESE MEDICINE
 by U Xiangcai

The Essential Guide to Understanding the Human Body

Synopsis: A light technical review of Traditional Chinese Medicine including some cause and effect of one's body problems.

1. Traditional Chinese Medicine (TCM) is a discipline that deals with human physiology, pathology, diagnosis and the treatment and prevention of diseases.

2. The theoretical system of TCM consists of the theories of yin and yang, the five elements - zang-fu organs, meridians, pathogenesis, syndrome and techniques of diagnosis.

3. The concept of wholism refers to a general view of the human body as a single, integrated entity that interrelates with nature.

4. Although yin and yang are opposites and oppose each other, they are also interdependent. Yin is installed in the interior of the body while yang remains on the exterior.

5. The practice of TCM medicinal substances are differentiated in four ways: Nature, Odor, Taste and Action. Their properties are their four pharmacological features, namely: cold, hot, warm, and cool.

6. TCM holds that the term qi refers to the essential substance that creates the human body and maintains its life activities. The physiological functions of qi include: impulsing, warming, defending, communicating, and regulating.

7. The nutritive qi and body fluids are regarded as the principal material bases for blood formation

8. Zang (viscera) refers to internal organs of the body, while xiang (appearance) refers mainly to the outward physiological and pathological manifestations.

9. The heart, lungs, spleen, liver and kidneys are together known as the five zang organs. The common physiological property of the five zang organs is to produce and store vital essence.

10. The heart performs two important functions: the maintenance of blood circulation and the control of vessel movement.

11. The spleen is located in the middle-jiao below the diaphragm. Its functions are to transport, transform, send up the nutrient, and to keep the blood flowing in the vessel. It is a chief organ of the digestive system.

12. If the spleen fails to regularly transport nutrients from food and thus fails to supply qi-blood, symptoms such as listlessness, weakness, dizziness, and loose stools develop.

13. The function of the liver is to store blood and regulate the volume of circulating blood in the body. When the liver does not supply adequate blood it effects the eyes, the tendons and may give rise to such symptoms as menorrhagia.

14. The main functions of the kidneys are: 1. To store essence. 2. To dominate growth, development and reproduction, and 3. To govern water metabolism and reception of air.

15. Deficient kidney-yin may lead to constipation due to dryness of the intestinal juice. Deficient kidney-yang promotes constipation or diarrhea due to disturbance in qi transformation.

16. The small intestine function is to temporarily store and further digest the partially digested food of the stomach and to separate the useful substances from the waste ones.

17. Marrow is classified into bone marrow, the spinal cord and the brain, all of which are manufactured by kidney essence.

18. The stomach dominates the receipt of food, while the spleen governs its transportation and transformation. The spleen transports the nutrients from the stomach for the rest of the body.

19. The Meridian Doctrine is the general term of both the channels and collaterals. The channel means the "route", and the collateral means the "network."

20. Du means governing and commanding. The du channel governs all of the yang channels of the entire body.

21. The twelve skin areas, where the qi channels disperses, are the areas that assist in the treatment and diagnosis of disease. This helps in diagnoses of the zang-fu organs via skin discoloration.

22. A disease is considered to be the outcome of the imbalance between yin and yang, organic trauma, and abnormality in physiological functions of the body.

23. TCM reveals the cause of a disease not merely by means of visual observation, but most importantly by analysis of symptoms and signs on the basis of clinical manifestations of the disease.

24. Pathogenic wind is the predisposing factor contributing to exopathic diseases. All the other pathogenic factors of cold dampness and dryness usually invade the human body in association with wind pathogen.

25. Since dampness is a pathogen that is yin in nature, an excess of yin may lead to disorder of yang. The syndrome (a group of symptoms which occur together) of arthritis is generally known as damp anthralgia (pain in a joint).

26. According to TCM the seven emotions refer to joy, anger, melancholy, meditation, grief, fear, and terror. They are emotional responses of the body.

27. Improper diet is often the factor predisposing to disease. Excessive nourishment due to overeating exceeds the ability of the spleen and stomach to transport and transform it and causes disease.

28. Phlegm retention is formed by an accumulation of water-dampness due to dysfunction of the lungs, spleen, kidneys, and resulting from invasion by the six exogenic pathogenic factors.

29. When blood stasis is formed, systemic or local circulation is hindered, thereby producing various syndromes.

30. Pathogenesis is the mechanism of occurrence, development and change of a disease. It is closely related to the strength of the body's qi and nature of the invading pathogenic factors.

31. After the onset of a disease its recovery or development depends on the outcome of the struggle between vital qi and pathogens.

32. Since qi bears a close relationship with blood and body fluid, deficient qi is bound to affect the generation, transportation, and distribution of blood and body fluid giving rise to many pathological changes of blood and body fluid.

33. Some of the clinical symptoms for deficient blood are: pale complexion, pale lips, dizziness, palpitation, lassitude and contraction of the joints.

34. Insufficient body fluid refers to a pathologic sate marked by dryness and resulting from a failure of body fluid to moisten and nourish the zang organs, pores, skin and hairs.

35. When blood is insufficient to nourish and retain heart-yang, the mind will not be nourished and mental activities are impaired.

36. Since the liver is an organ that stores blood, it is generally the first to be affected by an insufficient blood supply. Deficient liver blood leads to: malnutrition of tendons and vessels, restricted flexion of joints, and poor supply of blood to the head and eyes.

37. Diagnosticians use four techniques (inspection auscultation, olfaction, interrogation and palpation) to examine a disease's symptoms and signs, allowing them to determine the disease's causes, pathogenesis and most effective treatment.

38. Abnormal color and nature of stool may reflect pathologic changes in the spleen, stomach and intestines.

39. The voice is produced by the coordinated activities of the larynx, epiqlottis, tongue, lips, teeth, nose, and by functional activities of vital qi.

40. Cough is a manifestation of purifying and descending functions of the lungs leading to adverse rising of lung-qi. When listening to cough, focus attention on the sound of the cough and changes in amount, color, and quality of the sputum.

41. A foul smell like the odor of rotten apple from the mouth is attributed to diabetes.

42. When a balance of yin and yang occurs, an excess of yang leads to fever, whereas an excess of yin causes chills.

43. The head is the confluence of all the yang channels. In TCM the brain is referred to as the sea of marrow and is closely related to kidney-essence.

44. The best time for pulse-feeling is the early morning because the patient is then less affected by food intake and other activities. Qi and blood in meridians are less disturbed.

45. Pulse taking is made by pressing the arteries with the palm surfaces of three fingers. Strenuous exercise, emotional excitement, eating and drinking often cause the pulse to speed up.

46. Differential diagnosis of yin and yang is the general guiding principle underlying differential diagnosis. For instance, exterior, heat, and excess syndromes are yang, while interior, cold, and deficiency syndromes are yin.

47. The spleen's inability to transport or transform nutrients due to insufficient spleen qi is usually caused by: improper diet, fatigue, internal injury, or other acute of chronic disorders.

48. The retention of cold and dampness in the spleen is attributed to excessive cold and dampness in the body and impaired yang of the middle-jiao.

49. Deficient liver-blood is due to dysfunction in both the spleen and kidneys. Massive loss of blood or consumption of liver-blood is a cause of chronic disorders.

50. Deficient kidney-yang results mainly from kidney-dysfunction in the aged, kidney injury due to chronic disorders, and intemperance in sexual life.

51. Deficient spleen-qi usually results from: improper function of the lungs due to chronic cough with dyspnea, and injury of the spleen due to improper diet and overstrain. This leads to its failure to transport essence to the lungs.

52. TCM has always attached great importance to prevention. In Neijing, the concept of preventive treatment of disease before it actually happens is their belief.

53, To eliminate pathogens means getting rid of pathogenic factors to facilitate restoration of vital qi. Eliminating pathogens can be achieved mostly by using of purgative methods for excess syndrome when invasion by pathogens is the primary contradiction and vital qi has not yet declined.

54. When any of the zang-fu organs function inadequately, all of the other organs may be affected. The doctor must consider not merely the diseased organ alone, but also the interrelationship between all zang-fu organs.

55. Three conditions form the basis for the therapeutic principle by which an appropriated method of treatment is adopted: according to seasonal conditions, local conditions, and physique sex, and age of an individual.

30. PRIME TIME by Marc Freedman
How Baby Boomers will Revolutionize Retirement and Transform America

Synopsis: A look at how retirement has changed, and the many ways and organizations available to individuals so they can remain active mentally and physically in their retirement years.

1. The Work Connection inspired by Peter DiCicero was to get union retirees involved in mentoring kids and helping them break into the job marker. In the process, the retirees themselves gained a new lease on life.

2. What teenagers were saying was that they needed, more than anything else, adults who cared about them, who listened to them, and who were willing to take a personal interest in their lives.

3. The implications of an aging society have been primarily arbitrated by two groups of experts: physicians advising us on the exponential increase in dependency, disease and dementia of this fast-growing group, and financiers and economists who look to gain financial benefits.

4. Older Americans possess what everybody else in society so desperately lack: time. First, they have time to care. Second, they

have more time lived. Third, they have a longer time lift to live which may give them more reason to become involved with others.

5. Older adults are an untapped resource for society. Polls show that older people want to be more involved as shown that they vote at a higher rate than any other segment of the population.

6. There is one thing everybody seems to agree on: The boomers will not accept the old notions of later life and retirement. They will want to stay involved.

7. Retirement communities first started appearing in America in the 1920's. Organizations in Florida acquired land with plans to turn these plots into supportive living environments for their older members. However, the idea did not progress until after World War II.

8. The first community to bar residents from the younger and middle generations was Youngtown. Developed in 1954 it was just sixteen miles from the Del Webb Company's downtown Phoenix, Arizona offices. Del Webb planned its first Sun City in 1960 and now are in many locations across the country.

9. By the early twentieth century, maturing men and women were counseled to avoid the appearance of old age entirely, as thinning hair, false teeth, and failing eyes all were indicators of social uselessness.

10. The passage of the Social Security Ace of 1935 established a federal old age pension program. In 1940 payment of the first monthly Social Security benefits began. The Initial age was set at 65, at a time when life expectation was only 62.

11. Insurance companies were the first institutions to create formal retirement preparation programs.

12. The most conspicuous defining amenity at a Sun City retirement community was and still is golf. Golf courses make industrial-tract housing look more like paradise.

13. Since Sun City came into existence, leisure had become the defining ideal of retirement. By 1982, nearly half the new Social Security recipients retired in order to pursue leisured lives. However, one of the most disturbing trends from the Sun City idea is the rapid increase in gated communities.

14. Along with Medicare, launched as an amendment to the Social Security Act, the Older American Act was passed in 1965. This act was

set up to stimulate the development of community programs aimed at meeting the needs of the elderly.

15. The Foster Grandparents Program, which now involves over 25,000 older Americas serving 100,000 children, is based mostly in children's institutions, such as hospitals, orphanages and centers for the developmentally disabled.

16. The Foster Grandparent Program, launched by Lyndon Johnson, reveals that it is possible to create a national initiative recruiting older Americans to provide assistance to the younger generation.

17. Studies have shown that Foster Grandparents had more complex brain activity, better memory, and better sleep patterns than before they became involved in the program.

18. Volunteers in Medicine, a group started and available for those individuals who neither qualify for Medicaid or Medicare, nor have any private insurance, wanted to avoid any perception of being in competition with local practicing doctors.

19. The uninsured are finding that their last resort, charity care, is being threatened by the rapid expansion of managed care, which puts financial pressure on doctors and hospitals to focus their resources on insured patients.

20. The Samaritan House, where doctors and dentists donate their retired time, have two other key aspects: First, practice medicine for its value not as a business, and Second, they are involved in passing on this vision and motivation to the next generation of physicians.

21. The nation will need two million new teachers over the next ten years, with the larger gaps predicted in inner city schools. To help alleviate this potential problem, a bill was proposed called Troops to Teachers. It was designed to help men and women coming out of the service become certified as a teacher.

22. The examples of Volunteers in Medicine, Hope Meadows, and Troops to Teachers are just a few of the hundreds of new ventures aimed at reinventing retirement in a way that blends personal fulfillment with social renewal.

23. The conventional view is that society owes its older citizens something. But the organization Experience Corps volunteer group's view is that the older group owe something too and it is a sense of "operation give-back."

24. AmeriCorps, a domestic Peace Corps, was for older adults and the fastest growing group within the Peace Corps.

25. The author's hope was that we might someday turn our schools into "mentor-rich environments" where young people have opportunities to connect with a variety of caring adults during the school year. A pilot program was started by the Experience Corps in the most needy inner-city elementary schools

26. The number one reason individuals joined the Experience Corps pilot inner city school program was the concern of what was happening to children particularly the next generation of African American children overall.

27. In a study at Johns Hopkins it was found that the volunteers in the Experience Corps, 68% of the participants stated that they had learned new skills, while 74% said that they had grown personally.

28. The Wall Street Journal reported a sharp rise in the number of men in their fifties and sixties became physician's assistants after retiring. They were from a far different field from their work life.

29. A 1998 survey by AARP found that 80 percent of baby boomers were planning to work during their so-called retirement years, in contrast to 12 percent today.

30. Research at a Del Webb retirement community had revealed that boomers in their third age (retirement) will want state of the art fitness centers and new developments wired for the Internet, and not shuffleboard courts anymore.

31. There is a role for every sector of our aging population. That is fulfilling the aging opportunity and making America a good place to grow older, a place where third agers remain a vital and contributing part of society.

.

31. REMEMBER by Lisa Genova
The Science of Memory and the Art of Forgetting

Synopsis: A review of our brain and memory, and how we can lose memory to Alzheimer disease. Also included are ways how we can help to improve our memory.

1. We can often forget sometimes not because it's efficient for our brains to do so but because we haven't supplied our brains with the kinds of input needed to support memory creation and retrieval.

2. Creating a memory takes place in four basic steps: Encoding, Consolidation, Storage, and Retrieval.

3. The information contained within an experience that is collected by our brains is linked in a part of the brain called the hippocampus. It binds one's memories with other parts of your brain. If damaged, say by Alzheimer's disease, your ability to create new memories will be impaired.

4. If we want to remember something, above all else, we need to notice what is going on. Noticing requires two things: perception (seeing, hearing, smelling) and attention.

5. You can sustain the same information longer in your working memory by repeating it, either aloud or in your head.

6. Working memory is available in the present moment that captures your attention. It is sent to your hippocampus where it is consolidated into a long-term memory.

7. We have three types of long-term memories: memory for information, memory for what happened, and memory for how to do things.

8. Popular culture calls the ability to perform a previously learned skill Muscle Memory. This memory is developed through repetition and focused practice, where unrelated physical movements can be bound together and executed as a single action instead of a series of separate steps.

9. While semantic and episodic memories are consolidated via the hippocampus, muscle memories are bound together by a part of the brain called the basal ganglia.

10. The stuff you know, so-called Semantic Memory, is knowledge disconnected from any personal when and where. It is data unattached to any specific life experience.

11. As you progress from novice to master, brain scan studies show that the parts of your motor cortex activated by that skill become enlarged. Repetition is the key to muscle memory mastery.

12. Don't pull an all-nighter before a test. You are highly unlikely to remember this information next week or next year. Space out what you're trying to learn. You'll remember more and forget less.

13. The more emotional the event, the more vividly and elaborately detailed the memory. Emotion and surprise activate a part of your brain called the amygdala, which, when stimulated, sends powerful signals to your hippocampus.

14. Most of life's episodic memories are likely to be clustered between the ages of fifteen and thirty. This is called the reminiscence bump. These episodes are what we remember most in life.

15. How can we better retain our episodic memories: 1. Get off your routine, 2. Get off your devices and look up, 3. Feel it, 4. Repeat it, and 5. Keep a journal.

16. Every time we retrieve a stored memory for what happened, it's highly likely that we changed the memory. When we retrieve a memory of something that happened, we are reconstructing the story, not playing the videotape.

17. Writing something down allows you to rehearse and therefore strengthen the memory for the details you choose to remember about.

18. One of the most common experiences of memory failure is known as blocking or tip of the tongue (TOT). You know you know the elusive word or phrase, but you cannot retrieve it on demand. It's stored somewhere in your brain.

19. The frequency of TOT's we experience does normally increase with age, probably because of a decrease in our brain's processing speed.

20. Prospective memory is your memory for what you need to do later. This kind of memory is a bit like mental time travel and relies on eternal cues to trigger their recall.

21. To help prospective memory we can: 1. Make a to do list, 2. Enter the information into your calendar, 3. Use pill boxes for your medications. 4. Place your clues in impossible to miss locations.

22. Although information we encode into memory degrades rapidly with the passage of time, it doesn't entirely disappear. There are two main ways to resist the effects of time on memory: repetition and meaning.

23. Forgetting is quite important: it helps us function every day in all kinds of ways. It's advantageous for us to get rid of any unnecessary, irrelevant, interfering, or even painful memories.

24. We tend to think of remembering as the challenge but forgetting can be difficult, too. Motivated redirection of attention is a powerful way to ensure that an experience or information won't be retained.

25. Episodic memory recall decreases normally as we age. Writing down what you need to remember later is not a sign of weakness or cause for shame at any age. It's just good sense.

26. If you eat a Mediterranean diet, exercise regularly, meditate daily, and sleep for eight hours a night, you'll absolutely improve your memory performance in the near term.

27. Using strategies and insights as paying attention, decreasing distractors, rehearsing, self-testing, using visual and spatial imagery, and keeping a diary will improve memory at any age.

28. Although the molecular causes of Alzheimer's are still debated, most neuroscientists believe the disease begins' when a protein called amyloid beta starts forming plaques in our synapsis.

29. Alzheimer's begins in the hippocampus. The first symptoms of Alzheimer's are typically forgetting what happened earlier today or even moments ago. It is why people with Alzheimer' repeat the same story or question over and over.

30. Progression from the first symptoms of forgetting to end-stage Alzheimer's takes an average of eight to ten years.

31. Paying attention is the number one thing you can do to improve your memory at any age. A lack of attention will impair it.

32. The two workhorse stress hormones released by your adrenal glands are adrenaline and cortisol. Adrenaline is a fast-acting and short-lived emergency alarm. Cortisol is a little slower than adrenaline and mobilizes glucose (energy) so that you can physically respond to the stressful situation.

33. In a study, people under chronic stress are twice as likely to develop Alzheimer's disease as are people who are less stressed. While we cannot free ourselves from stress in our lives, we can train ourselves to become less reactive through yoga, a healthy diet, exercise, and meditation.

34. With respect to memory, sleep plays a critical role in many ways: 1. You need sleep to pay attention. 2. Sleep helps consolidate new memories. 3. Sleep optimizes muscle memory.

35. There is power in napping. Subjects who napped improved their pre-nap performance by 16 percent. The people who didn't nap showed no change in performance. A twenty-minute nap should be enough time to give you plenty of memory-boosting benefits.

36. Alzheimer's is caused by an accumulation of amyloid plaques. During deep sleep, your glial cells flush away any metabolic debris that has accumulated on your synapses.

37. Ninety-eight percent of the time, Alzheimer's is caused by a combination of the genes we inherited and how we live.

38. Both the Mediterranean and the MIND diets cut the risk of Alzheimer's disease by anywhere from a third to a half. These diets include green leafy vegetables, brightly colored berries, nuts, olive oil, whole grains, beans, and fish.

39. No studies show that drinking red wine reduces your risk of Alzheimer's. Anything that interferes with sleep increases the risk of Alzheimer's and this includes alcohol.

40. As a general rule, anything that is good for your heart is good for your brain and for preventing Alzheimer's.

1. FIGS, DATES, LAUREL, AND MYRRH
by Lynton John Mussenman

Synopsis: A review of many types of plants and their use in our daily life.

1. Trees are prominent in the Bible and biblical messages can be summed up by four trees: tree of life, tree of knowledge of good and evil, the tree that Jesus died on, and the tree of life in the last book of the Bible-Revelation

2. The leaves used on Palm Sunday are from the Date Palm.

3. The Dead Sea is located at lowest spot-on Earth below sea level-1319 feet.

4. Banana is from banan the Arabic word for finger.

5. The English word for line is from the Latin word flax- linum. Words such as linear and lineage are derived from the same linguistic root.

6. Frankincense is a gum from specie of the boswellia tree or shrub. It is dried to a resin. The word means high quality incense.

7. Poison hemlock should not be confused with the common tree in English as hemlock, which is not toxic and is used to make the original root beer.

8. The laurel tree is mostly known for its leaves - bay leaves. The family of these trees is also known for cinnamon.

9. Mulberry bush is where the silk worms make their silk.

10. Myrrh- is dried resin from the shrubs or small trees of the specie of Commiphora. There are two types- medicinal and fragrant, and from the Hebrew word mor.

11. Olives- oil has five main uses- food, illumination, ointment, soap, and preservative. It can be stored up to six years. Fresh olives are bitter if eaten off of the tree. They turn black when ripe. They are soaked in brine to remove the bitter taste.

12. Pine-seed for pine or pinyon nuts come from the stone or umbrella pine tree. Most know come from China. The pitch of pine trees was used for caulking on ships and sealing wine amphoras.

13. Pistachio, cashews, and mangos are in the same family as poison ivy. If allergic to poison ivy you may be allergic to these nuts.

14. Wheat is second most important plant after rice. All is used- the straw for bedding, basketry, roofing, and bricks. Each grain consists of

a minute embryo-germ, a large amount of starch-endosperm, and the fruit coat-bran. Three types of wheat are einkorn, emmer wheat, and durum. Barley is the main ingredient in the production of beer although wheat was used to a lesser extent.

15. Wormwood is used to flavor alcoholic drinks and known as absinthe or bitters.

2. Grain Brain by David Perlmutter

Synopsis: A review of bread and its elements, and its effect on our body.

1. Your brain weights about 3 pounds and has one hundred thousand miles of blood vessels.

2. Gluten is a "silent germ" and can inflect damage on our brain.

3. Pills focused on illness not wellness. This treatment of taking pills are often more dangerous.

4. A sugar level of 70-100 milligrams per deciliter is considered normal.

5. Brain disease for the most part starts with the diet. With too many carbs and too few healthy and unhealthy fats.

6. Insulin in our body escorts glucose into our cells. This promotes fat retention.

7. Type 2 diabetes is reversible through diet and lifestyle changes. There is no cure for Type 1 diabetes. Type 1 is known to be from genetic and environmental influences.

8. Diabetes jumped by 50% between 1995 and 2010, and 100% in 18 states.

9. High carb diet and gluten are the most prominent stimulators of inflammatory pathways that reach the brain for brain disorder.

10. High cholesterol reduces your risk for brain disease and increases longevity. High levels of good fat are proven to be key to health and peak brain function.

11. High blood sugar greater risk of brain shrinkage.

12. LDL is not a cholesterol (lipoprotein) and nothing bad about it.

13. Celiac disease is when an allergic reaction to gluten causes damage specifically to the small intestine.

14. Neuropathy is nerve damage outside the brain and spinal cord. Causes numbness, weakness, or pain.

15. Following are gluten free: buckwheat, quinoa, soy, and tapioca. Following contain gluten: beer, baked beans, blue cheese, bouillon, breaded foods, cereals, and chocolate milk.

16. Framingham Heart Study- associations between total cholesterol and cognitive performance.

17. Parkinson's disease strongly related to lower levels of cholesterol.

18. Heart attacks are affected at the same rate with either high or low cholesterol levels.

19. Consumption by individuals of highest amount of saturated fat had 19% lower coronary heart disease.

20. There has been no published study in the past 30 years to demonstrate that eating a "low-fat, low cholesterol diet" prevents or reduces heart attack or death rate.

21. Finding that it did not matter whether you ate large amount of fatty animal products or followed a vegetarian diet, the arterial plaque was the same in all parts of the world.

22. Gluten found in high-carbohydrate foods -pasta, cookies, cakes, bagels or whole grain bread, potatoes, corn, and rice.

23. When the American Diabetes Association recommended American should consume 60-70 % of calories from carbohydrates the rate of diabetes exploded.

24. Carbohydrates not dietary fats are the primary cause of weight gain. Farmers fatten their animals with carbohydrates like corn and grain

25. Human brain consists of more than 70% fat.

26. Certain vitamins like A, D, E, & K require fat to get absorbed. That is why we need dietary fat in our diet.

27. Vitamin K good for brain and eye health, and risk of age-related dementia and macular degeneration.

28. Vitamin D is an anti-inflammatory helping the body to get rid of infectious agents.

29. Side effects of statins- fatigue, shortness of breath, problems with balance and muscular pain and loss of coQ10 in muscles- reduced energy production.

30. Aerobic exercise turns on genes linked to longevity and brain's growth hormone.

31. 20% of our oxygen is consumed by the brain.

32. Cumin, the main ingredient in the spice turmeric (member of the ginger family), is good for the brain and good for detox along with green tea and coffee.

33. Coconut oil good for the brain and reduces inflammation.

34. Dark Chocolate with cacao above 70% is healthy.

35. U.S. is ranked #1 in the world in health-care spending and ranked 37th in overall health according to World Health Organization.

3. Meatonomics by David Robinson Simon

Synopsis: Some information on food and its relevance to people.

1. Animal agriculture drives one of the largest causes of climate change through greenhouse gases and more than transportation and power plants.

2. Since 1983 milk consumption has climbed 12% to 620 pounds per person per year mostly through promotions.

3. Teenagers consume 78% more saturated fat and 48% more cholesterol than suggested by the government guidelines. One in three teenagers is obese or overweight.

4. Per "The China Study" cancer is related to animal protein. Study shows that animal-based foods increased tumor development while nutrients from plant-based foods decreased tumor development.

5. Animal cruelty is against the law.

6. It is unlawful to defame food in a quarter of the U.S. states.

7. The 28-hour law where food or water must be served to animals do not apply to chickens or turkeys which account for 98% of all land animals killed for food in the U.S. This law does not apply to intrastate travel, which is exempt.

8. The cows treated with rBST insulin is a carcinogen and is banned in Canada, Australia, NZ, Japan, and most Europe though not in the US. Industry has stopped this through bills.

9. Two thirds of Government farming support goes to the animal foods that the government suggest we limit. Less than 2% goes to the fruits and vegetables it recommends we eat more of.

10. The USDA spent $30.8 billion in 2013 supporting US farmers with loans, insurance, research, marketing, cheap water, etc.

11. Farm subsidies were $161 billion between 1995 and 2009. The large farmers – big corporations got 9/10 of the cash. Two thirds did not receive a cent.

12. U.S. subsidized products like corn and soybeans provide ½ the products consumed on Earth. Most goes to third world countries hurting their ability to produce their own produce.

13. Study shows that mothers who ate large amounts of hormone implanted beef during pregnancy decreased fertility among those children. It is banned in most countries except the U.S.

14. One third of the food we eat depend on honeybee pollination. Their colonies decreased in half since 1945 related to GMO and pesticides.

15. Due to sport fishing and depletion of smaller fish, the salmon family is now ½ its weight and length. Also affected are bears and eagles.

16. Fish susceptible to parasites and live only in salt water. In fish farms they are removed from their salt water and infested with chemicals.

17. 95% of farmed fish that Americans eat is imported from regions like China and S. America.

18. 90% of agriculture workers lack health insurance, 1/3 are undocumented, 1/4 live in conditions that the state agency called "extremely overcrowded". At the Smithfield plant there is 100% turnover each year when 5,000 workers quit.

4. Omnivore's Dilemma by Michael Pollan

Synopsis: A review of corn its makeup and its use.

1. Corn comes from a single specie known as zea mays- a tropical grass. Everything we eat comes from and uses corn. From cows, corn syrup, chicken.

2. 40% of Mexican diet comes from corn via tortillas- maize or "walking corn".

3. Corn has 4-carbon atoms- C-4. 97% of what corn is comes from air and three % from the ground. From the air it gets its carbon through

its stomata or microscopic orifices in the leaves. A single corn seed yields more than 150-300 kernels. A wheat seed yields about 50 seeds.

4. Corn- eaten off the cob, ground into flour, brewed into beer or distilled into whiskey.

5. Maize is self-fertilized and wind pollinated. The tassel housed the male organs and yield about 14 million grains per plant.

6. The American Indians were the first to breed and develop corn for almost every environment. American corporate breeders figured out how to control the corn's reproduction so that the farmers had to buy new seeds each year.

7. Soybeans finds its way into 2/3 of all processed food via cattle, etc.

8. Corn in 1920 average about 20 bushels per acre about the same as the Indians.

9. Pesticides are based on poison gases developed for the war and now used by the chemical fertilizer industry.

10. Earth atmosphere is 78% nitrogen. More than half of the n2 is applied to corn. Corn now requires about 1/3 gal of oil to produce a bushel of fertilized corn today or 50 gal. per acre.

11. Corn has about 14% moisture.

12. Cargill and ADM buy about 1/3 of the corn in the U.S. and control the pesticide and fertilizer market, elevator, brokers, etc.

13. Cows normally eat grasses not corn. They have a separate digestive system called rumen to ferment the grass. Cows are now fast fed to grow in weight from 80 to 1,000 lbs. in about 14 months.

14. The modern coffee break began as a whiskey break called the elevenes.

15. Omega 6 is produced in the seeds of plants while omega 3 is in the leaves. Too high of 6 will contribute to heart disease because omega helps blood clot while omega 3 helps it flow. Hydrogenating oil eliminates omega 3.

5. The China Study by Colin Campbell

Synopsis: This study reviews the eating habits of the Chinese and its effect on their health.

1. Casein, which is 87% of cow's milk protein, promotes cancer. Least protein promoting cancer is from plants including wheat and soy.
2. People who eat the most animal food get the most disease.
3. One in 13 Americans has diabetes. We spend 1 of every 7 dollars on health. Other countries spend ½ what we spend and are healthier. U.S. is ranked 37 in the world on health
4. Proteins are a string of amino acids. They can all be derived from plant food.
5. Most all peanut butter is contaminated. With an AF (aflatoxin) factor of 300 times that judged acceptable by the US food.
6. Studies show nutrients from animal foods increase tumors while a decrease in tumor with plant food.
7. In US most of our calories of protein comes from animal food while in China a low % comes from animal food.
8. Coronary heart disease in very low in developing countries due to their high consumption of plant food.
9. People who eat the most animal protein have the most heart disease, cancer and diabetes.
10. The China study- people eating the most animal protein were taller and heavier, and had higher total and bad cholesterol.
11. China's cholesterol levels were between 70 and 170. Safe level should be about 150.
12. Framingham Study shows that we treat disease not prevent it. Diet not considered. Fat has 9 calories per gram while carbohydrates and protein have 4 calories per grams.
13. Only 3% of breast cancer can be attributed to family history.
14. Cancer Research- exercise helps to prevent colon cancer. Men with highest dairy intake had double risk of prostate cancer.
15. Only 5-6% dietary protein required.
16. None of the top 25 medical institutes teach nutrition. Of the billion plus budget only 3.6% devoted to nutrition. These budgets are for the development of drugs and supplements.
17. Hippocrates advocated diet to prevent and treat disease.

6. The Food Revolution by John Robbins

Synopsis: A study of food its laws, its use and affect.

1. U.S. spends nearly double on health care per capita than other leading countries as Germany, Canada, and France. Every 30 seconds someone in the U.S. files for bankruptcy for health problems.

2. Meat increases risk of diabetes and soy reduces the risk of hip fractures by 36%.

3. Livestock generates 65% of nitrous oxide gas and 18% of greenhouse gas emission higher that cars, shops and planes combined.

4. Blood pressure is lower among vegetarians.

5. Cancer Institute says being active, not smoking, and dietary items with plant-based foods can prevent most cancers.

6. Food basis- to prevent lung cancer- green, orange and yellow veg's- 40% reduction. The best items are carrots, sweet potatoes, yams, apples, bananas, and grapes. To help prevent prostate cancer for men- eat tomatoes. Stay away from meat, dairy and eggs.

7. The National Cancer Institute spends only $1million/year on promoting fruits and vegetable.

8. Annual medical costs in the U.S. –from meat consumption $100 billion, from smoking $65 Billion.

9. Best source of Calcium- brussel sprouts, mustard greens, broccoli, kale and all are about double that of milk.

10. Chickens – about 50% are contaminated with salmonella.

11. Penicillin discovered by Sir Alexander Fleming. Do to over use, some bacteria is now resistant to this drug.

12. Nearly half the water consumed in the U.S. is for livestock.

13. The Ogallala aquifer under S. Dakota to Texas is the largest body of fresh water on earth.

14. #1 milk producing area in the U.S. is Central California with only 4 water quality inspectors in Calif. Central Valley with 1600 dairies where the animals all contaminate the water supply.

15. About 2/3 of land In the central states from Montana to Arizona Is used for livestock grazing.

16. Last 35 years the Arctic Ocean ice thinned by 40%. 23 of the last 25 hottest days occurred after 1975.

17. First genetically engineered food sold in the U.S. was the FlavrSavr tomato by Calgene Corp now a sub of Monsanto.

18. Monsanto Corp founded in 1901 to manufacture saccharin.

19. Soybeans now are about 80% genetic and yield 4-10% less. It was initially touted for a greater yield.
20. Organizations that regulate genetically engineered crops and foods in the U.S.- FDA, USDA, and EPA.
21. Not required by law to advise the public that genetically engineered hormone is made from or included in a product as milk.
22. Global acreage planted to soybeans 54%, corn 28%, and canola 9%.
23. Monsanto has Roundup Ready for their genetic crops that the farmers must use by contract once they convert to their genetically modified products.
24. The only GMO potato is the Burbank Russet.

7. Consider the Fork: by Bee Wilson

Synopsis: Some interesting facts and information on items of cooking.

1. The word technology comes from Greek – Techne means art or skill and logia means study something.
2. Soft food tends to make you gain fat. Fibrous food has to do more work and energy in the body.
3. What has lips, mouths, necks, shoulders, bellies and bottoms- POTS. Pots became common about 10,000 BC in S. America and N. Africa.
4. Earliest recipes came from Mesopotamia (Iraq, Iran, and Syria) on three stone tablets about 4000 years ago.
5. First non-stick pans in France by Tefal Company in 1956. M. Gregoire, a French Engineer, developed PTFE.
6. First fires- striking pyrite rock against flint.
7. Thomas Edison first created a successful light bulb in 1897.
8. In 1795 France decreed a law to use liters, grams, meters (metric system).
9. Only three countries have not adopted the metric system- the United States, Liberia and Myanmar.
10. Cuisinart was launched in the U.S. 1973.
11. Mayonnaise- egg, table spoon of vinegar, two tsp of mustard, and salt and pepper. Put in bowl and wisk.
12. Why did Italy adopt the fork? - Pasta.

13. Chopsticks- Japanese are shorter at 22cm vs. Chinese at 26cm and have pointed ends.
14. Clarence Birdseye created the modern frozen food industry in the 1920's.
15. In 1930 50% of women were in paid work. In1950, it dropped to 34% and in 2000 it was 60 %.
16. Ergonomics- study of equipment that fits the limitations and abilities of the human body.

8. EAT MOVE SLEEP by Ton Rath

Synopsis: A review of helpful ways that anyone can improve their health and life by reviewing what they eat, how much they exercise and plan their sleep habits.

1. You can make decisions today that will give you more energy tomorrow. The right choices over time greatly improve your odds of a long and healthy life.
2. Researchers have estimated that 90 percent of us could live to age 90 with some simple lifestyle choices. The sum of your habits determines your life span.
3. Starting your day with a healthy breakfast increases your odds of being active in the hours that follow. For your overall approach to eating, avoid anything that is fried, consume fewer refined carbohydrates, and eat as little added sugar as possible.
4. Professor K. Anders Ericsson, found that elite performers need 10,000 hours of "deliberate practice" to reach levels of greatness. The best performers slept 8 hours and 36 minutes and typically practice in focused sessions lasting no longer than 90 minutes.
5. When you sit down, enzyme production, which helps breakdown fat, drops by 90%. After two hours of sitting, your good cholesterol drops by 20 percent.
6. Set a goal of eating foods that have a ratio of one gram of carbs for every one gram of protein. Avoid foods with a ratio higher that 5 to 1 carbs to protein.
7. Sugar is a toxin. Any packaged product with more that 10g is more than you need in a single serving.

8. Generally speaking, produce, with dark and vibrant colors, is your best bet as broccoli, spinach, kale, celery and peppers. Also look to red and blue fruits and vegetables.

9. Sleep deprivation raises blood pressure, increases inflammation, and boosts the risk of heart disease and stroke.

10. Based on the latest research, 10,000 steps per day is a good target for overall activity. This leads to significant health benefits.

11. Studies show that eating fewer carbs' curbs cancer growth rates by as much as 50 percent. Instead of chips, or bars for snacks select nuts, carrots, apples, celery, kale chips or seeds.

12. Exposure to light in the hours before you go to sleep suppresses melatonin levels. Lower melatonin levels make it hard to fall asleep and decrease sleep quality.

13. Onega-3s are essential fatty acids shown to protect against certain cancers, cognitive decline, macular degeneration, and heart disease. Ideal sources are fish, and nuts, seeds; salmon, walnuts, and flaxseeds are the best.

14. The epidemic of inactivity through technology spans the globe, from the United States to India and China.

15. Sleep less, achieve less. Surgeons and pilots now have mandated periods of rest before they are allowed to operate or fly an airplane.

16. It is easier to sleep in a dark, cool room than in a warm room. You have a natural body clock that regulates your core temperature.

17. When preparing your next few meals at home, use smaller plates. They found that a clear contrast between food and plate keeps people from overeating.

18. Regular exercise may be the best way to ensure a good night's sleep and more energy the following day.

19. An Australian study of more than 12,000 adults estimated that every single hour spent watching television after the age of 25 decreased the viewer's life expectancy by 22 minutes.

20. In one study, scientists found that the use of constant background noise can be remarkably effective at improving sleep.

21. Foods likely to increase the health and thickness of hair include blueberries, salmon, spinach, and walnuts. The key is to have an overall balanced diet with the right nutrients.

22. To prevent the growth and spread of cancerous cells in your body, consume more of these foods: apples, artichokes, blueberries, broccoli, kale, green tea, lemons, tomatoes and mushrooms.

23. Flavor ingredients that have cancer fighting potential: cinnamon, garlic, nutmeg, parsley and turmeric.

24. Studies suggest that regular exercise helps the cells inside your body sweep away debris, such as viruses and bacteria that accumulate over time.

25. When researchers study the exact amount of sleep people need to feel fully rested, they find that 95% of us need somewhere between seven and nine hours of sleep per night.

26. If you sleep less, you eat more. You remember less. You get sick more often, and can lead to high blood pressure.

27. Put it all together- eat right, move more, and sleep better.

9. THE FATE OF FOOD by Amanda Little
   What we'll Eat in a Bigger Hotter Smarter World

Synopsis: A review of how and where we get our food will be changing in the coming years.

1. The United States has been struggling not with a food deficit, but with calorie overload. Nearly 40% of our population is obese, and more than two-thirds are overweight.

2. As many as two billion people might not exist if it hadn't been for the advent of agribusiness. Farms globally now produce 17% more calories per person then they did in 1990.

3. In March 2014, the Intergovernmental Panel on Climate Change (IPCC) reported that droughts, flooding, invasive species, and increasing weather volatility were already hurting agricultural productivity worldwide.

4. The United States imports more than half of its fruit supply and about a third of its vegetables.

5. As farmers began to produce crops in volumes well beyond the needs of their communities, they became merchants for goods to other countries. By AD 700, Muslim traders had established the early foundations of the global economy.

6. The first major panic over global food supplies began to percolate in the late 1700's. Thomas Malthus announced in 1789 that food supplies could not keep pace with demand. This was mostly ignored until the mid-1840's, when famine swept parts of United Kingdom.

7. The invention of hybrid seeds combined with the arrival of chemical pesticides and fertilizers brought on the paradigm shift known as the Green Revolution.

8. Pests are evolutionarily adept at developing resistance to chemicals. This is the reason why, in the forty years between 1960 and 2000, pesticide use in the United States doubled.

9. Apples are heterozygous, meaning that the seeds generated by each fruit are genetically different from the fruit itself. Modern apple orchards use a cloning process to propagate the narrow range of apple varieties they grow.

10. More pesticides and fungicides are applied to apple orchards then to any other fruit crop. The average apple sold in the United States today has been in storage for six to twelve months before it reaches a store shelf.

11. Farm size has grown exponentially over the past half century while the number of American farmers has declined from more than 6 million in 1910 to 2 million today.

12. Every major agricultural company from Monsanto, Cargill and John Deere, had accepted climate science well before 2016. They've been building research divisions and product portfolios to address this impact.

13. For most farmers in the United States, water availability is their major limiting environmental factor.

14. Researchers at Washington State University successfully tested "nanocrystals" that can coat and protect fruit buds in spring to prevent frost damage.

15. The glaciers on Mount Kenya, Africa's second highest mountain, have been shrinking, Fewer than half of the sixteen glaciers that existed a century ago on the mountain remain intact today.

16. In 2012, the government of Kenya banned both the import and commercial cultivation of GMO crops.

17. About 90% of the corn grown in America is genetically modified.

18. By early 2017, about a fifth of all the lettuce grown in the United States had been thinned by a robot called LettuceBot. This robot was envisioned to be a weeder that could radically reduce the use of agricultural chemicals worldwide.

19. The use of herbicides on American farms began in the 1940's with the application of a toxin developed by chemists in World War II. Monsanto released the chemical under the brand name Roundup.

20. No-till farming locks carbon in the ground. Plowing releases, the carbon back into the atmosphere, while no-till keeps it sequestered.

21. Proprietary farm equipment software and hardware makes it nearly impossible for individuals to fix their own gadgets or machines. This makes them dependent on the manufacturer of the equipment for repairs. As is the case with Monsanto's system of locking farmers into its herbicides and seeds.

22. Drones, sensors and robots are part of a growing network of data-collection and devices that can feed detailed information to farmers about their crops.

23. In the late 1990's experimental concept of indoor farming called aeroponics began. This is growing plants in trays with their roots dangling in midair and are fed by nutrient rich mist. This system used about 95% less water than conventional agriculture.

24. In order to guarantee food production for their people, China purchased land in thirty-three countries including Brazil and Argentina. Growers in the U.S. have holdings in more than twenty-five countries.

25. Saudi Arabia imports 75% of its food.

26. With the population in the world expecting to reach 9.8 billion by 2050, a 33% increase from today, we'll need to grow our food upward as well as outward on a bigger scale.

27. Salmon are anadromous, meaning they're born in freshwater rivers and travel long distances to saltwater seas to feed before migrating back upriver to spawn.

28. Although fish species are declining across the globe because of overfishing the demand for seafood will grow at least 35% in the next two decades. This will lead to an increase of farmed fish.

29. Salmon are fish eaters but can be converted in wild fisheries to vegetarian by feeding them with the same nutrients and fats they normally eat.

30. Cloning cattle presents a huge potential cost advantage because identical carcasses could allow beef slaughter to become fully automated.

31. In 2015, Memphis Meats was the world's first start-up to grow meat in a laboratory using tiny samples of muscle, fat, and connective tissues taken from living animals.

32. Cellular meats, another alternative, represents one approach to waste prevention. It eliminates the waste associated with meat contamination and distribution.

33. The average American throws out more than a pound of food a day. Most of the food waste in the United States, about 35%, is generated by households.

34. About 20% of all the fruit and vegetables produced in Minnesota gets trashed because they don't meet narrow aesthetic standards.

35. Agriculture consumes 70% of the world's freshwater.

35. The Sea of Galilee and Israel's other natural fresh water sources are now so overdrawn that they can provide only 10% of the country's total water needs.

36. The U.S. Geological Survey has predicted that more than three-quarters of the U.S. Southwest will be in a state of severe drought by midcentury. The U.S. relies on this area's food production.

37. The United Nations predicts that by 2025 Egypt will approach a state of "absolute water crisis."

38. Recycled wastewater is the fastest-growing area in the water industry.

39. Countries in Africa and the Middle East have endured crippling droughts and living under severe climate stress than ever before.

40. Quinoa is an indigenous protein-rich superfood that has entered a modern renaissance. It became known as the "mother grain" of the ancient Inca empire in Peru. Quinoa also tolerates water scarcity and salty soil.

41. Edible algae is a growing area of research as a potential protein supplement.

42. People want assurances not just that there will be enough food for all of us to survive, but that our culinary traditions, including our fresh-food supply, will continue to live on.

10. EAT TO BEAT DISEASE   by Willian W. Li. MD
The new science of how your body can heal itself

Synopsis: A review of some foods that could help your body operate more efficiently. Included is a review of some technical factors for the workings of your body.

1. The study of blood vessels is called angiogenesis. Blood vessels are essential for health because they bring oxygen and nutrients to every cell in our body.
2. Only one in five medical school in the United States requires medical students to take a nutrition course.
3. The five defense systems in our body are: Angiogenesis (our blood vessels), Regeneration (stem cells maintain, repair and regenerate our bodies), Microbiome (bacteria defenders in our body), DNA protection (our genetic blueprint), and Immunity (defends our body's health).
4. More than 100 foods can enhance your body's ability to starve cancer and keep those tumors small and harmless. Some of these are: tomatoes, black raspberries, pomegranate, beer and cheese.
5. Inside your body are sixty thousand miles of blood vessels whose job it is to deliver oxygen and nutrients to keep cells alive.
6.   Neuropathies occur when the function of your nerves is compromised. This can lead to numbness or pain that ranges from mild to crippling.
7. Your diet can be used for disease prevention as well as to help aid treatment.
8. People in Asia who consume lots of soy, vegetables, and tea in their diet have a significantly lower risk for developing breast and other cancers. The soy can be in many forms as edamame, soymilk or tofu. Be careful of soy sauce as it is very high in salt.
9. Stem cells grow and maintain every organ in your body such as muscles, nerves, skin, brain and eyeballs.

10. Chemo and radiation do kill cancer cells, but they also demolish the healthy stem cells in the bone marrow.

11. We can avoid some risk to our stem cells by reducing our exposure to air pollution, tobacco, and alcohol.,

12. Loss of brain stem cells in implicated is the development of dementia. Foods and beverages can activate a person's own stem cells, boosting the body's capacity to regenerate and heal itself from within.

13. Prebiotics (dietary fibers) are nondigestible foods that feed the healthy bacteria in our intestines. Probiotic foods such as yogurt, sauerkraut, kimchi and cheese, bring their own bacterial contribution to our inner ecosystem.

14. When you hear the term human genome, it is referring to the complete collection of genes, made up of DNA, that are required to code for what your body needs over the course of your life.

15. There are many steps you can take to safeguard your immune defenses throughout your life. These include exercise, proper sleep, lowering and managing stress, and your dietary choices as cutting down on sugar and red meat intake.

16. The central command of the immunity is located in four body sites: your bone marrow, your thymus gland, your spleen and lymph nodes, and your gut. Your bone marrow produces almost all of the immune cells in your body.

17. The cells of the immune system are known as white blood cells.

18. Your immune system can be weakened by such items as cancers and their treatments, alcoholism, and obesity.

19. Celiac disease is an intestinal disorder, which has an immune reaction to gluten, a group of proteins found in wheat, barley and rye.

20. Angioprevention refers broadly to a health approach that includes using food, medicines, and dietary supplements. It helps keep the body's angiogenesis defense system (developing of new blood vessels) in a healthy state or balance.

21. Cooking tomatoes with the skin on help release the lycopene in the skin, which had been shown to potently inhibit angiogenesis. It is best cooked in olive oil.

22. The heart is a muscle that needs robust angiogenesis whenever its coronary arteries become clogged by cholesterol-laden plaques.

Some foods that help this situation are tomatoes, soy, broccoli, cauliflower, kale, fruits as red delicious apples, plums , berries and sea foods.

23. Tea is the second most popular beverage in the world after water. Green tea has been shown to reduce harmful angiogenesis and cancer growth, lowers blood pressure, improves blood lipids and restores immune cells.

24. Individuals over the age of 75, who drank one and a half to two beers per day were found to have a 60 percent reduction in the risk of dementia and an 87 percent reduced risk of being diagnosed with Alzheimer's disease. Another helpful drink is red wine, which is associated with cardiovascular benefits and anti-cancer activity.

25. Olive oil, especially extra virgin cold pressed, has shown to include compounds as antiangiogenic, anti-inflammatory, antioxidant and anticancer properties.

26. Nuts contain the potent antiangiogenic omeg-3. Some of these nuts are almonds, cashews and walnuts.

27. Consumption of foods as dark chocolate and coco power which contains bioactives called flavanols help lower incidence of death from cardiovascular disease.

28. Foods made with whole grain are healthier because it includes the grain's outer shell, which contains fiber, as well as the inner core that contains bioactive polyphenols.

29. Studies suggest that rice bran can protect your stem cells. The safest sources of brown rice are California, India, and Pakistan, which has about a third less arsenic than brown rice than other sources.

30. Chlorogenic acid is a powerful bioactive found in high concentrations in coffee, black tea, blueberries , peaches, fresh and dried plums and eggplants.

31. The hallmark of the Mediterranean diet is that it comprises of fruits, vegetables, whole grains, legumes, nuts, olive oil and fish. It was one of the first studies to show the link between saturated fat intake and heart disease.

32. A study in China showed that fasting can stimulate brain regeneration.

33. The data on cranberry and pomegranate juice show how powerfully our diet can influence our microbiome (microorganisms in

and about our body), which can in turn influence out immune response to cancer therapy.

34. One way to help our microbiome is to actually eat bacteria and improve our health defenses. The foods most prevalent are sauerkraut, kimchi (fermented is best), cheese and yogurt. A word of caution on kimchi as it is very high in salt.

35. When it comes to microbiome, cheese is good for your gut. Some cheese preferences are: Parmigiano-Reggiano, Camembert, and Gouda. Other products with helpful bacteria are yogurt, and sourdough and pumpernickel bread.

36. The guiding principles for taking care of your gut microbiome follow three basic rules: Eat lots of dietary fiber from whole foods. Eat less animal protein. Eat more fresh, whole foods and less processed foods.

37. Some other key foods affecting the microbiome: Apricots, black beans, cabbage, kiwi, lentils, red wine, kale, eggplant, and walnuts.

38. Vitamins A,B,C,D and E are the building blocks of DNA. They can be found in foods such as : Spinach, carrots, red peppers, lentils, navy beans, and mushrooms among other foods.

39. To assist in reducing your body's cellular aging one might consume nuts and seeds as they assist in growing your telomeres, which are part of your DNA.

40. Some of the foods that can help your immune defenses include: mushrooms, aged garlic, broccoli sprouts, extra virgin olive oil, chile peppers, blueberries and pacific oysters.

41. Most research studies on diet and longevity show that restricting your calories increases life span. One might skip breakfast or lunch a few days each week.

42. Purple potatoes, if you can find them, have been found to be antiangiogenic and that they can kill cancer stem cells. The anticancer effects are preserved whether they are boiled, baked, or cooked as potato chips.

43. There is evidence that whole grain, nuts, plant-based foods and fish can help prevent diabetes

44. When considering food, and your health and disease, there are five important caveats to keep in mind.: First, most of the studies are done using epidemiological research. Second, most of these clinical

studies on food and specific health outcomes involve relatively few people. Third, We are learning that every individual is different. Fourth, Remember that if you are currently battling a disease, you should definitely consult your doctor before changing how you eat. Fifth, The biggest reason is that there are no magic bullets that will ward off all disease.

11. FOOD FIX by Mark Hyman, MD
 How to Save Our Health, Our Economy, Our Communities and Our Planet- One Bite at a Time

Synopsis: This is a review of our food system from farming, related companies, how it effects the economy, the population, and how the pending problem can be ameliorated.

1. Professional health organizations must face the reality that Big Food has a long history of lobbying against public health, influencing public policy to the detriment of society, and manipulating scientific research.
2. Global per capita healthcare costs are one tenth that of the United States and the global obesity rates are lower as well.
3. GMO seeds are sold to farmers by four big Ag seed monopolies. The farmers who use these seeds can only buy them from these companies.
4. In the United States only 27% of cropland is used to grow food for humans, while 67% is used to grow food for factory-farmed animals.
5. Up to 40% of our food is wasted in areas such as transportation, in restaurants, in our homes, and sent to landfills. Food production and food waste are the third biggest emitter of greenhouse gases in the world, after the United States and China.
6. Our diet and our food system are by far the biggest contributors to the factors that have led to the epidemic of chronic disease.
7. Pay attention to your energy, weight, digestion, and health conditions. Your body will tell you what it likes. Some suggestions are: eat mostly whole plants, eat more foods with healthy fats, eat pasture-raised eggs, eat beans, stay away from most refined vegetable, bean, and seed oils. Stay away from GMO foods.

8. Because of the overweight or obesity problem, Chile managed to include an 18% tax on sugary drinks to the dismay of the food industry. The United States does not have a federal soda tax but thirty-three countries do.

9. In the last 50 years we have gone from spending 5% of our gross domestic product on healthcare to spending almost 20%.

10. the US has eight agencies overseeing the government's food-related policies. They largely work separately making their policies confusing and conflicting,

11. Seventy-five percent of the foods purchased with SNAP (food stamp program) are ultra-processed junk food. This could be fixed with policy changes by eliminating certain products from the purchase with these stamps such as sugary drinks. Change policies to encourage the purchase of healthy fruits and vegetables.

12. In 2017, more than 11,500 lobbyists registered with the federal government. Some were former politicians and political aids all to protect the goals of Big Pharma's, Big Oil, corporations and the food industry's profits at all costs.

13. Fast-food companies do not want to be sued, as were the tobacco and oil companies, for making people fat, sick, or diabetic.

14. In 2016 a bill was passed limiting your right to know whether GMOs lurk in your food. GMO foods require pesticides and herbicides. About 64 countries have laws mandating GMO labeling including China, Russia and 28 European Union countries.

15. Government subsidies enable lower prices for processed food by encouraging growing of food surpluses, while not supporting farming of fruits and vegetables. Apples are the only fruit or vegetable, other than corn, that receives significant subsidies.

16. President Obama signed into law the Healthy Hunger-Free Kids Act that mandated that schools provide healthier foods to their students. The program was rolled back by President Trump's administration.

17. Antibiotics are fed to livestock on factory farms. They are widely used in industrial agriculture to reduce the spread of nasty infections caused by overcrowding, filth, or other cruel conditions.

18. Before you believe a headline, ask yourself some important questions: First, who paid for the study, Second, does the story mention who funded it?

19. The Food industry is part of the story of structural violence, embedded in the political and economic organizations that hurt minorities, the poor and the food insecure.

20. It is a form of apartheid in which the poor and minorities live in areas that lack healthy food and have an over-abundance of fast-food outlets and convenience stores.

21. What may surprise some people is that government-guaranteed loan programs support fast-food outlets which are far more prevalent in poor communities of color.

22. Reforms are very difficult to put into effect given our current political environment. Campaign finance laws make corporations able to contribute literally billions of dollars to influence policy and elections.

23. The majority of cognitive dysfunction in kids can be linked to poor nutrition. Iron deficiency, which is common, can lead to lower dopamine function and impaired concentration.

24. Farmworkers and food workers are the largest sector of workers in America. Without farmworkers and food workers we wouldn't be able to eat.

25. When the Fair Labor Standards Act passed, which established the minimum wage, it excluded farmworkers and domestic workers from the most basic workers' rights.

26. Farm work is one of the most dangerous jobs in America due to the exposure to pesticides. Most other countries have banned the chemicals used in the United States. These chemicals are not regulated by the FDA for human safety but regulated by the Environmental Protection Agency.

27. In 2018 Monsanto's GMO seeds accounted for 90 percent of US corn, 91 percent of cotton, and 94 percent of soybeans grown.

28. According to a 1992 agricultural census report, small diversified farms produce twice as much food per acre than large conventional farms.

29. Due to the use of pesticides, GMO, and poor farming practices on large farms, we have only about sixty harvests left from our soil to continue growing crops on our farms as we do today.

30. Eighty-five percent of subsidies go to 15 percent of the largest farms. More than 88 percent of our agricultural production comes from only 12 percent of farms.

31. Experts say we have globally lost 50 percent of our topsoil. Soil degradation is caused primarily by livestock overgrazing, industrialized agriculture, deforestation, over fertilizing, tilling, and bad crop rotation.

32. We are witnessing a massive insect population collapse due to pesticides and land use changes. We have seen a 75 percent decline over 30 years in flying insect biomass.

33. A large study of farms using regenerative or sustainable practices shows that they are actually more productive than agrochemical-dependent farming practices.

34. Policies needed for a saner approach to our agriculture and food system would be: Establish a national food policy, increase funding research on sustainable agriculture, end the ethanol mandate, consider a "nitrogen tax", and ensure the next farm bill helps break up monopolies of farm seed and agrochemical companies.

35. Industrial agriculture contributes to climate change through the overproduction of the three main GHGs (greenhouse gasses): methane, nitrous oxide, and carbon dioxide. The top five suppliers emit more GHGs than oil companies do.

36. We need to build systems that can address regeneration of soil, water, climate, biodiversity and human communities.

12. THE CASE AGAINST SUGAR   by Gary Taubes

Synopsis: This is a review of the effects of sugar and the disease it could causes in our body through reports of studies throughout the world. These diseases include diabetes, tooth decay, obesity, high blood pressure, high triglycerides, and heart disease.

1. Fifty years ago, one in eight American adults was obese. Today the number is greater than one in three and about one in nine is diabetic.

2. In 2019, one in seven to eight adults in the United States had diabetes. Among U. S. military veterans, one in every four patients admitted to VA hospitals suffers from diabetes.

3. Anywhere populations begin eating Western diets and living Western lifestyles, diabetes epidemics tend to follow.

4. During World War I, with the government rationing and sugar shortages, diabetes mortality invariable declined.

5. The term sugar refers to a group of carbohydrate molecules of carbon, hydrogen and oxygen. They refer to glucose, galactose, dextrose, fructose, lactose, and sucrose. Sucrose is composed of equal parts of glucose and fructose.

6. As for tobacco, sugar was and still is a critical ingredient in the American blended-tobacco cigarette, The first of which was Camel.

7. In a study published in 1952, agronomists could get cattle to eat plants they otherwise disdained by spraying the plants with sugar or molasses.

8. In 1920 during Prohibition, sugar consumption in the United States hit record highs, while breweries were being converted into candy factories.

9. The sugar plant is technically a grass, growing to heights of twelve to fifteen feet, with juicy stalks that can be six inches around. Within a day of cutting, the sugarcane stalks will begin to ferment and then rot, thus the need to immediately process.

10. It was Columbus who first brought sugar to the New World on his second voyage in 1493.

11. From the seventeenth through the nineteenth centuries, sugar was the equivalent, of what oil was in the twentieth century.

12. Two factors drove the final transformation of sugar from a luxury for the wealthy to a pleasure for all: it was the development of the beet-sugar industry and the other was the transformation of sugar into a dietary staple via technology. Four industries emerged: candy, chocolate, ice cream and soft drinks.

13. Ice cream consumption doubled between 1940 and 1956. Now sugar would become a mainstay of breakfast as well, first in fruit juices and then in sugar-rich breakfast cereals.

14. Indulgence of sugar has exceeded every other stimulant, even including tobacco, coffee, tea and alcohol.

15. IN 1924, Medical Associations considered the increase in sugar consumption that paralleled the increasing prevalence of diabetes to be the prime suspect. In a 1971 text, physicians and nutritionists around the world began to suggest that sugar was an obvious cause of obesity, diabetes, and now heart disease.

16. When blood-sugar (glucose) levels rise, the pancreas secretes insulin in response, which then signals the muscle cells to take up and burn more glucose.

17. Observation has shown that the obese had high blood sugar and high insulin levels.

18. In 1940, when the military draft began, 40 percent of the first million men called up for service were rejected for medical reasons, the most primary one was extensive tooth decay.

19. John Yudkin wrote in 1963 of the situations in England- "Sugar provides about 20 percent of our total intake of calories and nearly half of our carbohydrates."

20. In a research study, Yudkin had subjects fed sugar-rich diets and reported that this raised both their cholesterol and their triglycerides.

21. The two items that tracked best with heart disease were sugar and saturated fat.

22. The French had relatively low rates of heart disease despite a diet that was rich in saturated fats. It was realized that the French consumed far less sugar than did the Americans and British.

23. The Sugar Association proclaimed that "Sugar does not cause death dealing diseases. "

24. In the 1980's, the public health authorities in the U. S. were telling Americans that fat was what made them fat and implying that sugar was effectively harmless as long as we didn't overdo it.

25. Insulin resistance and a condition now known as "metabolic syndrome" (a host of disorders that were thought of as unrelated as high blood pressure, high triglycerides, and heart disease) is a major, if not the major, risk factor for heart disease and diabetes.

26. Short-term studies suggest that a high-fructose intake consisting of soft drinks, sweetened juices, or bakery products can increase the risk of metabolic and cardiovascular diseases.

27. How and why diabetes and obesity could explode throughout Native American people: 1. Change in diet and lifestyle by

Westernizing, 2. Sugar seemed to be the prime suspect as they became insulin-resistant, 3. Genetics are also involved.

28. A research reported that 45 percent of the children of diabetic mothers had become diabetic themselves by the time they were in their mid-twenties.

29. The evidence for sugar or fructose as a primary cause of gout is twofold: 1. The increase as the population becomes Westernized, 2. The fructose component of sugars increases serum levels of uric acid.

30. In the mid-1960's the pharmaceutical industry developed an inexpensive drug called allopurinol that could lower uric acid levels to prevent future attacks of the gout disease.

31. In 2003 in a published analysis in the New England Journal of Medicine reported that cancer mortality in the United States was clearly associated with obesity and overweight.

32. If the sugars we consume - sucrose and HFCS (High Fructose Corn Syrup) specifically cause insulin resistance, then they are prime suspects for causing cancer as well.

33. Alzheimer's, like cancer, is associated with type 2 diabetes, an observation that began to emerge from studies in the mid-1990's.

34. In the type-2 diabetes disorders, perhaps the high blood sugar (glycemia) is responsible for the increased risk of Alzheimer's disease: the higher the blood sugar the greater the oxidative stress in the brain.

35. If sugar causes insulin resistance, and thus the type 2 diabetes and the hypertension, then sugar also increases the likelihood that dementia is in our future.

13. . FAST FOOD NATION   by Eric Schlosser
The Dark Side of the All-America Meal

Synopsis: A review of the growth of the fast-food industry including its chains, its food sources, and the food laws.

1. On any given day in the United States about one-quarter of the adult population visits a fast-food restaurant. Today about half of the money used to buy food is spent at restaurants- mainly at fast food restaurants.

2. The McDonald's corporation is the largest owner of retail property in the world. It earns the majority of its profits not from selling food but from collecting rent.

3. The fast-food chains demand for a uniform product have encouraged changes in how cattle are raised, slaughtered, and processed into ground beef.

4. In late 1944, Carl Karcher owned four hot dog carts in Los Angeles. When a restaurant across the street from the Heinz farm went on sale, he bought it and changed it into Carl's Drive-In Barbeque.

5. At the end of the 1940.s the McDonald brothers closed their drive-in restaurant. They got rid of everything that had to be eaten with a knife, spoon, or fork and adopted the principle of factory assembly line into a commercial kitchen. This encouraged Karl Karcher to open his own self-service restaurant

6. Twenty-five years ago, only a handful of American companies directed their marketing at children,- Disney, McDonald's , candy makers, etc. Today most companies are doing just that. They learned that brand loyalty may begin as early as the age of two.

7. Studies of the fantasy lives of young children suggest that until the age of six, roughly 80 percent of children 's dreams are about animals and thus the start of clubs as Disney's Mickey Mouse Club.

8. A ban on children's advertising was proposed but it was attacked by the National Association of Broadcasters, the Toy Manufacturers of America and others.

9. Facing revenue shortfalls, in 1993, District 11 in Colorado Springs started a nationwide trend. It became the first public school district in the United States to place ads for Burger King in its hallways an on the sides of its school buses.

10. Fast food chains benefit when children drink more soda. Soda has by far the highest profit margins. In 1978, the typical teenage boy in the United States drank about seven ounces of soda every day. Each can contains the equivalent of about ten teaspoons of sugar and most contain caffeine.

11. The American School Food service Association estimates that about 30percent of the public high schools in the United States offer branded fast food.

12. More than 70 percent of fast-food visits are "impulsive." Brand loyalty follow these visits.

13. McDonald's Corporation has used Colorado Springs as its test site for its restaurant technology, as software and machines designed to cut labor costs and serve fast food even faster.

14. About two-thirds of the nation's fast-food workers are under the age of twenty. The fast-food industry seeks out part-time , unskilled workers who are willing to accept low pay. Although Franchises must obey corporate directives , they are not covered by federal laws that protect employees.

15. Worker instructions are made very simple written at a fifth-grade level and written in Spanish and English

16. The industry has benefited with government tax credits which they claimed up to $2,400 for each new low-income worker they hired. This helped subsidize the industry's high turnover rate which has been about 300 to 400 percent per year.

17. Managers try to make sure that each worker is employed less that forty hours a week, thereby avoiding any overtime payments.

18. The heart of a franchise agreement is the desire by two parties to make money while avoiding risk. The franchisees sacrifice a great deal of independence by having to obey the company's rules. It was the fast-food industry that turned franchising into a business model soon emulated by retail chains throughout the United States.

19. During the 1990's , Subway was involved in more legal disputes with franchisees than any other chain. They have about fifteen thousand restaurants, second only to McDonald's. It costs about $100,000 to open a Subway restaurant, the lowest investment in any major fast-food chain.

20 . French fries did not become well known in the United States until the 1920's. Do to its size and high starch content the Russet Burbank was the perfect potato for frying. Once bought frozen it became the most profitable item on the menu.

21. The taste of a fast-food fry is largely determined by the cooking oil. Originally McDonald's cooked its fries in 7 percent cottonseed oil and 93 percent beef tallow. After much criticism, the oil was changed in 1990 to vegetable oil with added "natural flavors."

22. Man-made flavor additives were used mainly in baked goods, candies and sodas until the 1950's, when sales of processed food began to soar.

23. The growth of the fast-food chains encouraged consolidation in the meatpacking industry. McDonald's is the nation's largest purchaser of beef.

24. The top four meatpacking firms are: ConAgra, IBP, Excel, and National Beef. They slaughter about 84 percent of the nation's cattle.

25. Twenty years ago. Most chicken was sold whole, today about 90 percent of the chicken sold in the United States has been cut into pieces, cutlets, or nuggets. In 1992 American consumption of chicken for the first time surpassed the consumption of beef.

26. About half of the nation's chicken growers leave the business after just three years, either selling out or losing everything.

27. Most American beef cannot be exported to the European Union, where the use of bovine growth hormones has been banned.

28. The meatpacking giants have cut costs by cutting wages. They have turned one of the nation's best paying manufacturing jobs into one of the lowest-paying, creating a migrant industrial workforce of poor immigrants. All this responding to the demands of the fast food and supermarket chains.

29. In 1961, the Iowa Beef Packers opened its first slaughterhouse-a meat factory. The labor principles followed that of the McDonald brothers and designed a production system for their slaughterhouse in Denison, Iowa. This eliminated the need for skilled workers.

30. The Reagan administration did not oppose the disappearance of hundreds of small meatpacking firms, on the contrary, it opposed using antitrust laws to stop the giant meatpacker.

31. The slaughterhouse is one of the nation's largest. About five thousand heads of cattle enter it every day, single file, and leave in a different form. Meatpacking is now the most dangerous job in the United States.

32. Once a slaughterhouse is up and running, fully staffed, the profits it will earn are directly related to the speed of the line. A faster pace means higher profits.

32. When Ronald Reagan was elected president in 1980 OSHA was under staffed but the OSHA inspectors were still cut by 20percent. At that point the number of serious injuries rose.

33. Every day in the United States, roughly 200,000 people are sickened by a foodborne disease. Today the U.S. government can demand the nationwide recall of non-food items but it cannot order a meatpacking company to remove contaminated ground beef from fast food kitchens and supermarket shelves.

34. Dairy cattle can live as long as forty years, but are often slaughtered at the age of four, when their milk output starts to decline.

35. The McDonald's chain earns the majority of its profits outside the United States, as does KFC. McDonald's now ranks as the most widely recognized grand in the world, more familiar than Coca-Cola. The chains try to purchase as much food as possible in the countries where they operate.

36. Fast food is the one form of American culture that foreign consumers literally consume. The United States now has the highest obesity rate of any industrialized nation in the world.

37. The fast-food industry has made an abundance of high-fat, inexpensive meals widely available. Thus, leading people to eat more meals outside the home while consuming more calories, less fiber, and more fat.

38. In 1948, The first In-N-Out Burger was opened on the road between Los Angeles and Palm Springs. It was the nation's first drive-through hamburger stand. The owners declined to sell the chain and refused to franchise it. It pays the highest wages in the fast-food industry and is ranked the first in food quality, value, service and cleanliness.

39. Congress should create a single food safety agency. Currently the two main organizations USDA and the FDA have separate tasks.

40. McDonald's has stopped serving genetically engineered potatoes as they were doing in Europe.

PLANT SECTION

1. For All The Tea In China by Sarah Rose

Synopsis: A review of the tea plant and how it was located in China, and secretly taken and replanted in other countries.

1. Tea was first introduced into England in the 1880's.

2. Tea was grown on the Himalayan's in Indian in the Assam Province in the 1815.

3. Plants can survive for years kept in a sealed, well-lit environment without water.

4. The East India Company hired 'Robert Fortune a Biologist to go to China to discover their source of tea and bring it to India.

5. Lilac came for Persia, tulip from Turkey, citrus from Southeast Asia, camellias from China, cinchona from Peruvian to produce alkaloid quinine.

6. Mexico received independence from Spain in 1821.

7. In China, Robert Fortune learned:

     a. Green tea leaves were left exposed to the sun for one to two hours to dry. They were then put into a wok and cooked to break the cell walls down. Then put on tables and crushed by rolling with bamboo poles.

     b. Green and black tea leaves come from the same plant. Black leaves are fermented while green tea is not. Leaves sit in the sun an entire day to oxidize. This treating produces the tannins- bitter taste and dark color.

     c. To the green tea the Chinese added two pigments- Prussian blue- Ferro cyanide and a yellow substance calcium sulfate dehydrate (gypsum). This was mixed with the green tea because the English wanted it to look green.

     d. Black tea needs sugar, as it is bitter while green tea does not.

8. Leaves are picked from April to October from each bush every 10 days. The best leaves are the small ones from the top of the bush. Each picker mostly female carry two bags each up to 60lb's.

9. Tea is easily cloned by cutting any branch and replanted, left to sprout and will develop a network of roots. This process is called gamogenesis.

10 For centuries China had forbidden its people access to the ocean even to fish.

11. Slavery ended in Britain in 1833, as they could no longer find workers for its sugar colonies.

12. The first mass-produced mass marketed global commodities were sugar, coffee, tobacco and opium.

13. British defeated Napoleon in 1815 and they then did not need the expensive warships.

14. The Suez Canal was built and completed in 1869 by the French due to the heavy traffic from Far East trade to save sailing time around   Africa.

15. Per pound black tea has more caffeine than coffee but contains half the caffeine as coffee by the cup because one pound of tea brews about 200 cups while a pound of coffee yields barely forty cups. Green tea has about 1/3 the caffeine as black tea.

16. Caffeine is a chemical alkaloid, a base, and stimulates the nervous and cardiovascular systems.

17. Black tea takes sugar and green tea does not.

18. Plants can survive for years kept in a sealed well-lit environment without water.

19. Queen Elizabeth granted royal charter to the East India Company in 1600. They bought spices and fabrics from the Orient and sold them in London. They hired Fortune to investigate the tea of China. Once discovered he hid plants and returned to India to replant them

2. Teaming with Nutrients by Jeff Lowenfels

Synopsis: A review of plants and their needs to remain healthy.

1. 17th century Jean Helmont proved that plants actually didn't need fertilizers only water. Pulverizing soil particles makes them more edible to plant roots.

2. Plant cells size can be related to a period where five to fifty cells would fit into this area.

3. Polysaccharide fibers inside cell walls have a negative charge and attract positively charge particles known as cations.

4. Plasma is matter in a phase that can be in solid, or liquid or gaseous state or all three.

5. Phospholipids are two-part molecules with its head a negatively charged phosphate ion that is water-soluble.
6. Cytoplasm is all the stuff inside the cell membrane except for the nucleus.
7. DNA- deoxyribonucleic acid and RNA- ribonucleic acids are the molecules replicating the genetic code used to build everything in a cell.
8. There are about 10,000 different kinds of proteins in each microscopic cell.
9. Nutrients form 3 types of bonds: covalent, ionic, and hydrogen bonds.
10. Water can dissolve more elements than any other liquid. This is due to the hydrogen bonds, which is a great solvent.
11. Carbohydrates are carbon-based molecules- carbon, oxygen and hydrogen. It includes sugars, starches and cellulose.
12. Water moves in side roots by the xylem system that is three forces- transpiration, water cohesion and eater adhesion.
13. Stomata are leaf pores that open during the day to let in the carbon dioxide needed to make sugars.
14. All plants need a mere 17 of the 90 naturally occurring elements. There are 27 other elements but these are man-made and not required for plant survival.
15. Seaweed contains 60 natural elements.
16. Hydrogen, oxygen, and carbon make up 96% of the mass of a plant.
17. Earth's atmosphere consists of 78% nitrogen and 21% oxygen
18. Chlorophyll includes four nitrogen atoms and without these atoms there is no photosynthesis. Lawn's yellow due to a lack of nitrogen for making chlorophyll green pigment.
19. Lack of calcium leads to malformed plants especially in new roots, shoots and young leaves.
20. Lack of magnesium in plants show that the leaves start to lose their green color in between the leaf veins.
21. Sulfur deficiency first appears in younger leaves when they start to yellow. This yellowing could also be a symptom of low iron
22. Silicon helps cucumbers and roses grow.
23. Maize plants transpire about 4 gallons of water per week.

24. Tree rings give a record of precipitation and temperature in the past. As rains dissipate and the temperatures go up this increases transpiration and thinner tubular rings are developed.

25. Guttation is when water is mixed with tree sap and accumulates in the xylem cells. They then expand pushing the xylem sap up the plant where there is less pressure.

26. If a plant loses leaves you do not want to give it much water because the roots need to adjust to the lower number of leaves they are feeding.

27. The pH of phloem saps is usually alkaline between 7.5 and 8.5. 90% of compounds in sap are sugars.

28. Soil pH can lock up nutrients making them unavailable to plants.

29. Temperatures effect on plants. The mycorrhizal fungi are most active between 41-95 degrees. They are responsible for much of the plant's phosphorus uptake.

30. Micronutrients become less available as pH increases and only sulfur is not affected by pH.

31. Cation exchange capacity (CEC). These nutrients, if needed, should be added when they won't leach away from rains.

32. Chemical fertilizers have about 60% nitrogen content whereas organic fertilizers have about 12% nitrogen. Arthropods as mites and worms shun synthetic fertilizers. Mycorrhizal fungi are the largest single source of carbon in soils.

33. Pollution runoff from farms and gardeners from 32 states and two Canadian provinces enters the Mississippi River and flows to the Gulf of Mexico. In the spring the pollution causes huge algal blooms to form. When the algae dies they sink to the saltier water below, decompose and uses up the limited oxygen creating dead zones in the area where no fish can survive. Cooler weather in the winter disrupts this cycle for the time being.

34. Human hair- for every 7 pounds there is around 1 pound of nitrogen and is a good natural fertilizer.

35. Important to test your soil every 2-3 years to determine what nutrient it needs. Good nutrients can be supplied with cut grass, vegetables, annual flowers, etc.

3. The Drunken Botanist by Amy Stewart

Synopsis: A review of various plants and foods where they originated from and their use in conversion to other items as alcohol.

1. Agave is not a cactus but of the asparagus family. First drink made from the sap of this plant was pulque. The flowering stock is cut before it starts to form. Sap flows from this cutting. One plant can produce 250 gallons of sap. These plants only bloom once and then die.
2. Tequila, if standard, it is made up of 49% non-agave sugars. To be 100% agave it must be from Weber Blue with no sugar added and must be bottled by the producer in Mexico. Gold tequila is flavored, colored, and aged in oak barrels. Tequila was named by Franz Weber in 1890's.
3. Apples- contains more genes than humans. Cider is inhospitable to bacteria.
4. Yeast-eats sugar to form ethyl alcohol and carbon dioxide. At about 15% alcohol the yeast die.
5. Grains are packed with starch to make alcohol. The starch must first be changed to sugar and to do that you just add water.
6. Beer- Barley is one of the main ingredients. It originated in the Middle East then to Spain, China, and brought to the America's by Columbus on his second trip. It's what makes the foam in beer. There are two and six row barleys. The two rows have the most starch and the best for a higher alcohol level.
7. Kentucky produce 90% of the world's bourbon supply. Must contain at least 51% corn. Straight bourbon is aged at least 2 years with nothing added. Blended must contain 51% straight bourbon and other items.
8. Vermouth- made from white wine and fortified with brandy to about 16% alcohol. Red vermouth is just made with red grapes.
9. Potato traces its ancestry to Peru. Vodka first made in Russia and Poland, and made from grains. Vodka is made from sugar beets, grains, apples, grapes and acorns. Potato was made into vodka because of cheap source in Poland during the war. But all insist that the best is made from rye or wheat.
10. Sweet potato is a vine related to the morning glory and not a potato at all. Native to South America.

11. Sugarcane originated in New Guinea. Used as building material in some cases or the early shoots were just picked and chewed. Columbus brought it to the Caribbean where it flourished. This gave us slavery in the 1500's because of the hard work to produce sugar. Today 25% of the world's sugar comes from beets. In the United States this figure is 55%.

12. Aloe is related to agave plant and asparagus.

13. Artichoke- shown to protect the liver and lower cholesterol levels.

14. Clove is a tightly closed flower.

15. Gin is redistilled vodka with juniper and other items to add flavor.

16. Star Anise - 90% of the world's production is purchased by drug companies to make Tamiflu a drug to combat the flu.

17. Vanilla- native of Mexico. It is difficult to cultivate, as its roots need to be exposed to air that is called epiphyte. Its vines climb trees. One flower per day, over 2-month period, awaits pollination by a single species of stingless bees.

18. The chamomile flowers-are used for anti-inflammatory drugs.

19. Hops in beer help to make the foam. Beer is mostly make from barley and other grains and flavored with hops. It also preserves it and adds the foam from its lupine resin that contains acids.

20. Beer bottles are brown because light makes the liquid taste skunky. Something in the hops breaks down to cause this.

21. Roses strengthen the stomach and the liver.

22. Saffron- it takes 4 thousand flowers to get an ounce of saffron.

23. Cinchona tree- source of quinine extract.

24. Cinnamon- it is from the bark of a tree native to Sri Lanka. The best comes from there but also comes from India and Brazil. Cassia cinnamon sticks are thick and form a double roll while true cinnamon look like a tightly rolled bunch of thinner bark. True cinnamon comes from Ceylon. It helps liver problems.

25. Eucalyptus tree's oil is good for mosquito repellant.

26. Jefferson encouraged replacing sugar grown from canes with slave labor with sugar from maple trees, which required fewer slaves with less energy.

27. Grapefruit appears to be the hybrid of sweet orange and pomelo.

28. Meyer lemons- hybrid of a lemon and mandarin orange.

29. Lemon is a cross between lime, citron and a pomelo.

4. How Plants Work by Linda C-Scott

Synopsis: A study of plants their content, their care, and their development.

1. Tannins were named for early use in tanning leather. In wine or green bananas, a dry taste mouth. This binds your salivary proteins.
2. Flower colors- birds see best in red, bees in blue and are signs of pollination guides.
3. Vitamin B1 stimulates new root development and reduces shock. However, plants make their own B1 so adding it does nothing.
4. Gibberellins regulate plant height and development.
5. To ripen green tomatoes put them in a bag with a ripe banana. The ethylene released from the banana will transform the rock-hard tomatoes into a soft and juicy one.
6. Overwatered plants tend to turn the lower leaves yellow due to release of ethylene from stressed soaked roots.
7. The tree green cambium under the bark is the growth factor to elongate the tree.
8. Mycologists is the study of fungi. Endo means inside and ecto means outside when used with words. The roots of fungi limit disease and root pests.
9. Soil sulfur deficiency causes yellowing in plants. Phosphorus is needed for constructing membrane and is almost always in the soil.
10. Gypsum is calcium sulfate an inorganic fertilizer. Don't add nutrient to soil without knowing if it needs it as it could have a negative effect on plants.
11. Hydrangea colors of blue and pink are partially due to aluminum content.
12. Never add phosphate fertilizer to bulbs, groundcovers, perennials shrubs or trees unless testing shows it's needed.
13. Green chlorophylls and orange carotenoids trap photosynthesis. The color you see is the wavelength light that is not absorbed by the object.
14. Plants use the sun's energy to transform carbon dioxide and water into sugar and oxygen- that is photosynthesis. $6CO_2 + 6H_2O = C_6H_{12}O_6$ (SUGAR) $+6O_2$

15. Water moves to where water isn't. Red leaves have anthocyanins in cellular water and means less water than green leaves. It is harder for water to evaporate from red tissues.

16. Browning on the tips and edges of leave is an indicator of drought stress.

17. Plants close due to phenomenon called nyctinasty from the Greek words for night and pressing close. Plants measure time to close at night and open during the day by the light and the color reflections.

18. Some plants as rhododendron leaves are thermonastic. When temperature falls to freezing thy droop and curl to save heat. They open when the temperature increases.

19. Tropic from the Greek word to turn. Plants and trees follow the sun.

20. Heliotropic means follow the sun as sunflowers whereas paraheliotropic avoid the sun by keep their leaves parallel to the incoming sunlight.

21. Ausins cause the shadiest side of plants to grow the fastest. This causes trees to bend away from the shade and most leaves will be found on the least shaded side of the plant.

5. The Botany of Desire by Michael Pollan

Synopsis: This book is based on some history and facts of four plants, for their sweetness, beauty, intoxication or control. These plants are the apple, tulip, marijuana and potato.

Apples- fruit

1. Johnny Appleseed (John Chapman) planted apple orchards from western Penn. through central Ohio and into Indiana.

2. Edible apple plants had to be grafted otherwise the apples were sour. Cider was the fate of most apples up until Prohibition.

3. The apple industry came up with the slogan "An apple a day keeps the doctor away". This was to keep the government from demanding that apple trees be cut down during Prohibition.

4. Seed facts: seeds contain cyanide, and each is genetically different from one another called heterogosity.

5. Each apple has about 5 seeds.

6. They are said to have come from Kazakhstan.

7. Eating apples were the invention of grafting by the Chinese about 2000 BC.

8. Apples are the second most popular fruit after the banana.

9. Hard cider from apples is from their fermentation that converts the glucose to ethyl alcohol and carbon dioxide. Corn liquor was popular before the sweeter hard cider.

10. There about 2500 varieties of apples.

<u>Tulips- flower</u>

1. Honeybees favor radial symmetry to daisies and clover while bumblebees prefer the bilateral symmetry of orchids, peas and foxgloves.

2. The more perfect the symmetry of the flower the healthier and sweeter the flower.

3. Ogier Ghislain de Busgecq of Austria claimed to have introduced the tulip to Europe by sending a consignment of bulbs from Constantinople in 1554.

4. The word tulip comes from the Turkish word for "turban".

5. It takes 7 years for a tulip from a seed to flower and show its color.

6. The black tulip is called "Queen of the Night".

7. Each tulip has six petals in two tiers. The three inner petals are smaller and have a cleft top while the outer ones form uninterrupted ovals.

8. The tulip crash came in the winter of 1637.

9. Flora, the Roman goddess of flowers who was a prostitute famous for bankrupting her lovers.

<u>Marijuana -drug</u>

1. Compounds called flavonoids change the taste of plants on the tongues of certain animals.

2. Coffee was discovered by Abyssian herders in the 10th century observing that animals became frisky after nibbling on the shrub berries.

3. Peruvian legend discovered quinine by observing sick cats were restored to health after eating the bark of the cinchona tree. Catnip contains a chemical called. "Nepetalactone".

4. Most marijuana smoked in the U.S. was grown in Mexico until the mid-1970's when the Mexican government at the request of the U.S. to spray the crop with the herbicide paraquat to help eliminate the crop. The product could easily be identified because it grew to 15 feet tall with purplish green leaves.

5. Search for a type that grew shorter was found in Afghanistan that rarely grew taller than 4-5 feet.

6. The earliest known religion was the cult of Samoa who ate the intoxicant of the Amanita Muscaria, a mushroom sometimes called "fly agaric".

7. Marijuana is known to alter parts of the brain as the cerebral cortex (inner thought), hippocampus (memory), basal ganglia (movement) and amygdale (emotions).

8. Nietzsche said "they are the power of forgetting" consist in a kind of radical editing or blocking out of consciousness everything that doesn't serve the present purpose.

<u>Potato-vegetable</u>

1. The New Leaf potato was genetically engineered by Monsanto Corp. It produces its own insecticide.

2. The Colorado potato beetle was the scourge of the plant and ages the leaves overnight.

3. Ireland in 1588 almost everything grew poorly. The potato seemed to be the best to grow and with milk was a complete nutritious diet because it provided protein, and vitamins B, C, & A.

4. In 1845 from America to Europe arrived spores of a potato fungus.

5. The potato famine was the worst catastrophe to befall Europe since the Black Death of 1348.

6. Ireland depended on only one kind of potato, the Lumper that was not resistant to a potato blight. When the blight started it destroyed all the potatoes in Ireland.

7. The Incas and other societies in South America grew multi crosses of potatoes so that no one blight could destroy the entire crop.

6. Herbal Antivirals by Stephen H. Buhner

Synopsis: Looking at various plants and how they can effect various diseases and your health.

1. Plant-based medicines, unlike pharmaceuticals, don't cause resistance problems and are biodegradable and renewable.
2. West Nile enciphalis virus emerged in the United States in 1999. It then spread throughout the world.
3. Polio was unknown but by 1910 the disease swept the world. The Salk vaccine was discovered in 1955 to eliminate the disease. The vaccine was licensed for use worldwide in 1962.
4. DNA and RNA are living organ cells. DNA is a double-stranded molecule and RNA is a single-stranded molecule.
5. Estimates are that the Earth contains 10 to the 31rd power of viruses. Viruses have no nucleus and no cell wall. They live in the hottest and coldest parts of the earth.
6. Viruses, thought to be conquered, are making a comeback due to genetic rearrangements via learned resistance to antivirals.
7. The 1918 influenza pandemic was the most deadly plague that human beings ever experienced. It started as the 1918 war was ending and lasted until December 1920. It killed some 17 million people.
8. Neuraminidase inhibitors as Tamiflu are effective in the treatment of influenza. They inhibit the ability of the virus to enter host cells. Other natural neuraminidase inhibitors are: Chinese skullcap, elder, licorice and ginger among others.
9. Glucose during influenza infections significantly increases viral load and illness parameters.
10. Plant medicines, unlike pharmaceuticals, don't develop resistance to viruses.
11. Ginger is useful for the flu only if the juice of the fresh root is used.
12. Zinc and selenium are very helpful during influenza infections.
13. Parainfluenza viruses generally cause what is called croup. It is an acute infection of the upper respiratory tract accompanied by barking cough. Herbs specific for this are Chinese skullcap, elder and licorice.
14. West Nile virus first occurred in 1999 in the Americas.

15. Keeping melatonin levels high will reduce, or eliminate, the ability of the West Nile and other encephalitis viruses to cause infections.

16. There are two types of herpes: simplex virus 1 (HSV-1) –cold sores, and simplex virus 2 (HSV-2) – of the genitals.

17. Shingles sometimes leads to postherpetic neuropathy. Pharmaceuticals don't heal the disease but help with the episode and pain. Over-the-counter analgesics are often used. For treatment one can use zinc sulfate cream.

18. Plant and root, as Chinese skullcap root tinctures, are high in melatonin and can help with sleep.

19. Flavonoids improve memory dysfunction and reduce neuronal damage.

20. The elders contain high levels of phosphorus, vitamins A, B6 and C, and most of the amino acids. It has been in European medical practice for over 2,500 years treating inflammatory conditions.

21. Ginger has been cultivated for over 4,000 years in China and India. The plant is perennial, likes warm and humid climates, and is cultivated like potatoes. It is one of the most heavily cultivated plants on Earth.

22. It is estimated that up to half of all Chinese herbal formulas contain Ginger.

23. The herb isatis is used as a digestive tonic and for GI tract problems.

24. Licorice is potently antiviral and moderately antibacterial. It acts by inhibiting the ability of enveloped viruses to fuse with host cells.

25. Monolaurin is one of the major constituents of coconut oil. It has been found to be active against measles and other viruses including HSV-1 & 2.

26. Astragalus has been found effective in alleviating fatigue in heart patients and in athletes.

27. Rhodiola has been found effective in the treatment of breast cancer and found to be highly antioxidant.

28. Prior to WWII pharmacists were extensively trained in every sophisticated forms of herbal medicine making; this is why they are still called "chemists."

7. The Hidden Life of TREES by Peter Wohlleben

What They Feel, How They Communicate

Synopsis: A history and education of trees and how they grow, eat and survive.

1. Trees communicate through electrical impulses that move at about one third of an inch per second. Their path is through the soil web fungi.

2. Forests are superorganisms with interconnections much like ant colonies.

3. Trees and plants can distinguish between their own roots from the roots of other species.

4. Trees also communicate by scent. Acacia trees give off a warning gas to neighboring trees when being eaten.

5. Cultivated plants lose their ability to communicate to protect themselves from prey as pests. This is the reason why modern agriculture uses so many pesticides.

6. To "girdle" a tree is to remove a strip of bark 3 feet wide all around the trunk to kill the tree. This removes the cambium or green portion under the bark, which supplies water and food to the tree.

7. Beech or oaks pollinate by having the wind blow their powdery pollen out of the blossoms and carries it over to neighboring trees.

8. Willow trees are both male and female. Bees collect pollen from the bright yellow blossoms that attract the bees first. They then pollinate the female blossoms.

9. Young trees, offspring of the mother trees, grow slowly due to the canopy that lets only about 3% of the available sunlight reach the ground to the young tree.

10. Mature beech trees can send more than 130 gallons of water a day coursing through its branches and leaves. This water is needed for its food production. The tree stockpiles water in winter or the dry seasons.

11. Cambium is the life-giving layer under the bark of a tree. Remove the cambium from around the tree and the tree dies for lack of food and water. It is stuffed full of sugar and minerals. People can eat the cambium in case of an emergency.

12. The tree roots grow fine hairs that tap into damp ground to suck up as much water as possible.

13. Fungi's cottony web in the ground is more like insects. They cannot photosynthesize and depend on organic connections with other living beings they can feed on.

14. The delicate fungal fibers ward off all intruders, including attacks by bacteria or destructive fellow fungi.

15. Some fungi are "host specific" as birches and larches. Others as chanterelles get along with many different trees: oaks, birches, and spruce.

16. Some birds, such as the woodpecker, benefit the trees that become infected with insects as beetles. This helps the tree live.

17. Water makes its way up the tree from the soil by capillary action and transpiration. The narrower the vessel, the higher the liquid can rise against gravity. Suction is created when the tree exhales gallons of water a day.

18. The water pressure in trees is the highest shortly before the leaves open up in the spring. This is the only time of year you can harvest the coveted syrup from sugar maple trees.

19. Every year, a tree in its prime adds between 0.5 to 1 inch to its girth.

20. Trees stop growing taller when their roots and vascular system cannot pump water and nutrients any higher. The tree then starts getting wider.

21. Some trees have a defense against attack by insects and fungi. The oaks wood contains tannins. When oak barrels are used in making wine it is called "oaked" wine.

22. Spruce trees store essential oils in their needles and bark, which act like antifreeze in the winter.

23. Trees have a trunk and branches, and grow steadily upward. Otherwise, the plant is classified as a shrub, which has many smaller trunks or branches.

24. The tree roots are its brain. The root network is in charge of all chemical activity in the tree.

25. As trees photosynthesize, they produce hydrocarbons that fuel their growth. The forest is really a gigantic carbon dioxide vacuum that filters out and stores this component of the air.

26. The older the trees, the more quickly it grows.

27. Spruce trees are comfortable in low temperatures. Their branches are horizontally or slightly angled downward to lean on each other for support when the snow piles up.

28. The farther inland you go, the drier it is, because the clouds get rained out and disappear. When you get about 400 miles from the coast, it is so dry that the first deserts appear.

29. The foam that sometimes forms in pools after heavy rains is the result of humic acid, come from the decomposition of leaves and dead wood and are extremely beneficial for the ecosystem.

30. A forest with tall trees contains animals and insects (ants, aphids, etc.), fungi, and bacteria and exhales oxygen during the day.

31. Mycelium (white underground threads or roots of mushrooms) force their way into the roots of firs, beeches, oaks, and other species of trees.

32. A plant that isn't green doesn't contain any chlorophyll and, therefore, cannot photosynthesize. These plants rely on other plants for food.

33. Wood fibers conduct sound particularly well, which is why they are used to make musical instruments such as violins and guitars.

34. The more species there are around the less chance there is that a single one will take over to the detriment of the others.

35. A fifth of all animal and plant species depend on dead wood.

36. Trees like bears hibernate. Their leaves turn red shutting up shop for the year. The storage space under their bark and in their roots are full to shut down for the winter.

37. Mistletoes sticky seeds are deposited on tree branches when thrushes clean off their beak on the upper branches on a tree. Their roots then grow into the tree bark.

38. Moss species hold on to trees with their hair like structures and get their food from the exterior of the tree as water and dust.

39. Pioneer species, ones that are away from their mother trees, hate shade. Shade slows their upward growth and a tree that grows slowly has already lost.

40. Trees that produce heavy fruit as oaks and chestnuts rely on the animal world for their seed disbursement.

41. Trees exhibit great tolerance for variations in climate. The native European beech grows in Sicily as well as southern Sweden.

42. In the normal storm months from October to March, deciduous trees are mostly naked and offer little wind resistance preventing damage.

43. Deciduous trees don't catch fire from lighting because their wood doesn't contain any resins or essential oils. Cork oaks' thick bark protects them from the heat of grass fires.

44. After the ice age, trees moved into habitats where they found conditions that suited them. Each specie has habitats where they are happy to grow.

45. Leaves falling into streams and rivers leach acids into the ocean that stimulate the growth of planktons, an important part of the food chain